# Live Your Life

# Forget the Diet

# Find Your Zen

## Kenny Glover

Live Your Life, Forget the Diet, Find Your Zen

© 2017 Kenny Glover

# Dedication

God is always first in my thanks for education, ability, and inspiration.

Mom and Dad have always supported each and every creative endeavor throughout this journey of living.

Thank you sweet Kink and Bell, my wonderful puppy dogs, for always showing me love, understanding, loyalty, and making me a priority.

# Preface

The journey to write this book began 30 years ago. At 15 my body stopped growing and my metabolism ground to a halt. The understanding of my metabolism, daily exercise, counting calories, and finding a balance of mind, body, and spirit is an ongoing process.

Throughout my life, I have tried starvation and grapefruit diets to lose weight. Joined a gym to focus on training and aerobic exercise. Bulked up with a creatine supplement and my trainer Tina. Obsessed over how many kick boxing, cardio funk, and bench aerobic classes could be fit into a week. Wondered why it was so easy to gain weight and so hard to lose it. Walked on a treadmill and by myself around a track. Rode the yo yo of fitting into clothes, and having nothing to wear.

Life always fell into two states of being: I was losing weight or had just lost weight. There was no daily living. Enjoy it while you are slim until all the weight is gained back. Re motivate to lose it all again. This was a never ending cycle.

There has to be a way to eat, live, play, and be happy. A way to get off the roller coaster of losing and gaining weight. The pinnacle of this was after the passing of my father from Alzheimer's. The round the clock care for several months caused my weight to balloon up to 286. This was the heaviest I had ever been. To move forward, the weight had to be lost.

During this period of losing 50 pounds in 7 months, I began to put together a lifetime of experience, mistakes, and knowledge. Three years later, I find myself able to stay off the roller coaster and able to be in one state: *Live Your life, Forget the Diet, Find Your Zen.*

There are still challenges, obstacles, and a need to motivate one's self daily.

Throughout this journey, I have been a professional photographer, desktop publishing specialist, graphic designer and writer.

**To view my photography, background, and contact information please visit my sites:**

kenny-glover.pixels.com

Instagram: kennyglover1969

amerikanpie.com

Facebook: KG Image Solutions

kgfindyourzen@gmail.com

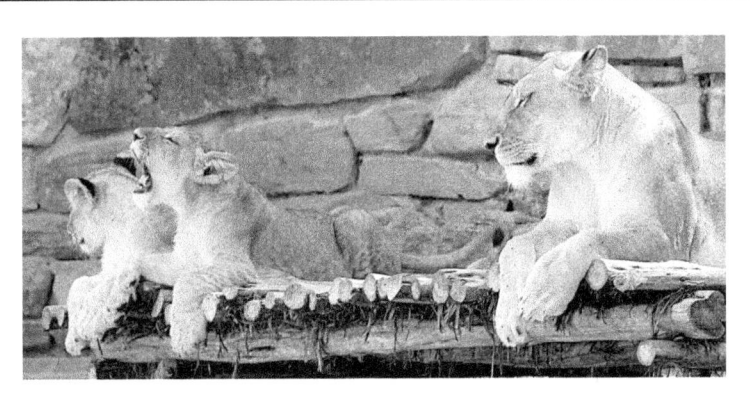

Lioness and cubs relax at the Ft. Worth Zoo.

This photo is available in any format at:

kenny-glover.pixels.com

# Contents

# 1 Getting Started

*Live Your life, Forget the Diet, Find Your Zen:* Sounds simple enough doesn't it? Contrary to what the billion dollar diet industry would have everyone think, maintaining a goal weight and living a healthy life style **is not** rocket science, found in a bottle, the latest fad diet, or new age exercise equipment.

The word **diet** conjures up a definition in our head: limit myself to small amounts of special kinds of food to lose weight. Every new diet comes with a new name. The result is the same. You are expected to follow their plan to achieve weight loss. There in lies the problem. Each person is different. If we are all different, how can one plan work for all of us?

The reality is it cannot and only works for those individuals whose parameters fit that particular plan. Then what? If it works, how long can a goal weight be maintained once living everyday life resumes? Living everyday life and maintaining a goal weight requires creating your own plan.

## How do I create my own plan?

1. To have a plan, there must first be a goal.

2. The goal needs to be achievable and realistic.

3. What is the motivation for my goal?

## Goal

We all know what weight is a good weight for our own body. A weight where you look good and feel well. A weight where the clothes you want to wear fit. This weight cannot be determined by a chart, index, or a trainer.

It is ultimately the weight that will make you comfortable in your own skin.

# Reality

There can never be a goal that is too big to reach. Sometimes the goal exceeds our grasp. It's like climbing a mountain. The first time out the goal is not the summit. The goal is the first overlook on the trail. Start out with a number that would make you happy and that is attainable. It may not be the final destination weight but, it is the first overlook on the trail. Be realistic by not putting a time frame on reaching this goal. That's the problem with other people's plans; there is an expectation especially when spending time and money to see results quickly and definitively. The reality is to *Live Your Life, Forget the Diet, Find Your Zen* start with a realistic achievable weight loss goal even if it's only 5 pounds.

# Motivation

This would seem to be fairly easy to define. Is it for your job, your spouse or mate, societal pressure, ego, vanity, desire to attract a partner, or any of a number of possibilities? The core motivation needs to be the ability to be content in your own skin. In essence, to like what you see in the mirror. Any other motivation will change when the circumstance or mood changes. Once the motivation changes so to will the ability to maintain a healthy, happy weight.

# Start Up the Trail

Now that there is a goal that is realistic and attainable and we are properly motivated, it is time to acquire the skills and equipment needed to reach that first overlook. It is time, step by step, to create a plan that will allow you to live everyday life and be happy and healthy in your own skin. Let's get started with the plan!

# Plan

1. Understand that weight loss is about biology and math.

2. Understand that weight loss is about cutting calories.

3. Learn how to count calories.

4. Download Fat Secret App.

5. Buy a good digital scale and decide how often to weigh.

6. Determine your average daily calorie consumption.

7. Figure out why you are eating?

8. What time of day are you hungry?

9. What's your kryptonite?

10. What's your yearly cycle?

11. Learn how to cut calories and eat same foods.

12. Create a meal plan or follow our suggested recipes and meals.

13. Learn to shop for fresh, healthy, and happy foods.

14. Find your Zen when it comes to exercise.

15. The relationship between exercise, counting calories and a goal weight.

16. Be a part of the natural world.

17. Find a balance in life between mind, body, and spirit.

18. How do I maintain?

19. What if I backslide?

# 2 Understand Weight Loss

Losing weight is about **biology** and **math:**

Biology of our bodies is simple. Eat more calories than you burn on a daily basis and gain weight. Eat less calories than you burn on a daily basis and lose weight.

Math is simple: 3500 calories = 1 pound

3500 / 7 days = 500 calories per day

Consume 500 less calories per day to lose 1 pound per week.

What drives the consumption of calories is metabolism. This is the process by which food is converted into the energy the body needs to function each day.

The number of calories the body requires to carry out the basic functions of living each day can be called the basic metabolic rate. This rate is determined by body size and type, sex, and age. The basic metabolic rate accounts for about 70% of daily calories. How the body processes food and the amount of physical activity accounts for the rest. The total calories consumed and the amount of physical activity are completely under each person's control. [1]

Even if you have inherited a slow metabolism, there are many things that can be done to increase the body's metabolism: [2]

1. Daily exercise

2. Strength training that adds muscle mass

3. Eat fish rich in Omega 3's - salmon, herring, and tuna

4. Do not drop below 1350 calories a day for women and 1500 for men or the body will start to burn muscle rather than fat because it has gone into starvation mode.

5. Enjoy **EPOC** throughout the day. This is the phenomenon known as **excess post** exercise **oxygen consumption**. It may take hours for a body to return to it's resting metabolic rate after an intense workout. Starting and finishing the day with exercise can only aid in increasing caloric burn during times of the day when the body might be sedentary.

6. Eat something for breakfast everyday.

7. Discover low calorie snacks to keep from being hungry throughout the day.

8. Think protein. It takes the body longer to process protein so you feel full longer and your body will expend more energy processing a high protein diet.

9. Cut trans fats which in processed foods are "partially hydrogenated oils". Trans fats slow down the body's abilities to burn fat and ultimately slow metabolism. Examples could include doughnuts, cookies, muffins, pies, cakes, commercially fried foods and baked goods made with shortening or partially hydrogenated vegetable oils.

10. Drink alcohol in moderation as it slows down the bodies metabolism and the calories are "empty calories".

11. Add cinnamon to enliven the meal and speed up metabolism.

# Conclusions

To lose one pound a week, 500 calories must be cut from the daily regimen. How fast and how many calories our individual body burns is based on our own metabolic rate. This rate can be increased over time aiding in weight loss and maintenance. It is important to note that starvation or extreme calorie cutting will only make the situation worse as the body burns muscle instead of fat and ultimately lowers the body's metabolic rate.

Note that muscle weighs twice as much as fat. Gaining a half pound of muscle per week and losing a pound of fat will result in no change on the scale. Based on what Zen you decide on for exercise, there will be two methods for measuring weight loss. Ultimately, the goal is to lose body fat. If strength training is not for you, then progress will be seen on the scale. If strength training will be part of your Zen someone will need to measure your body fat on a regular basis and body measurements will need to be taken for comparison to see whether progress has been made. This is the first important decision. If the validation of seeing the scale drop is motivation, then strength training can be added at a later date.

Different people add muscle mass at different rates. If you put muscle mass on easily then, any exercise may add muscle mass. For me, adding muscle mass was easy and the scale would go up even though I was losing body fat. Ultimately, it's going to be about finding your Zen and strength training will either be something you enjoy or a means to toning up. When I had a trainer at lunch, I used to enjoy training in the gym. Now, years later, my Zen is walking my dogs.

The most important thing is to: *Live Your life, Forget the Diet, Find Your Zen.* The easy path to success is the best way to start your journey. The path may be cutting 250 calories a day and getting 15 minutes of exercise until you lose your first five pounds. The exercise can be any enjoyable daily physical activity.

We will examine the tools and the knowledge needed to begin the path to a healthy, happy body image.

# **3** **Counting Calories**
## Tools / ADCC

Counting calories starts with understanding product labels.

**Each Label will list:**

**Serving Size** - A portion designated by the manufacturer. This may be the entire package or any of a number of units of measure from grams, tablespoons, cups, pounds, ounces, or even a certain number of pieces.

**Servings Per Container -** This number designates how many servings in the specified serving size are in the entire package.

**Calories -** This number represents the number of calories in 1 serving.

For example let's say you are going to have a pot pie for dinner. This is a normal pot pie intended for one person to eat. The serving size should be one pot pie. Careful, it's not. There are two servings in one pot pie. Reading the label in the store 410 calories seemed reasonable. When in actuality, the total calories for 1 pot pie is 810 calories.

Serving Size: 1 Half Pot Pie

Servings Per Container: 2

**Calories: 410**

This is what manufacturers want the consumer to think. They try to make their product seem as appealing as possible while still falling within what's required and allowed on the product label.

Calories: 820 is not printed on this label. What catches your eye is the **Calories: 410** in bold print.

The **first good habit** to fall into is to read the label of every product and know the calories per serving, servings per container, and how many servings you would normally eat during a meal.

# Serving Size / Portion

If you don't know how to convert a serving size into something that can be measured easily then, it will be a struggle to count calories. Let's get started with some basic measurements.

One tablespoon is not a heaping tablespoon. *If the serving size is in tablespoons, use a tablespoon to portion out the serving.*

For example foods like mayonnaise, peanut butter, chicken salad, salad dressing, and ketchup would normally be portioned out using a knife or straight from the bottle but, to get an accurate calorie count use a tablespoon.

1 tablespoon of ketchup is 20 calories - How many calories in a squeeze?

2 tablespoons of peanut butter is 190 calories - How many calories in a knife glob or heaping tablespoon? How many calories in what you licked off the knife?

*Conversion is the next issue.* Let's use chicken salad as our example.

Serving size: half cup

Calories: 320

Are you going to use a measuring cup to make a sandwich? No. Are you going to need a half cup of chicken salad to make two sandwiches? No.

Convert: **1 cup = 16 tablespoons**

1 half cup = 8 tablespoons

320 / 8 = 40 calories per tablespoon

Two tablespoons per sandwich only totals 160 calories for 2 sandwiches.

*What about foods that are poured into a bowl like milk and cereal?*

**Here's my trick:** Use a bowl that holds one cup of cereal as your cereal bowl.

Use a measuring cup to portion out 1 cup of cereal. Discover which bowls in the cupboard will hold a cup. A cup of milk will fill in the space in the bowl holding your cup of cereal. One cup of cereal and one cup of milk is a good serving size for a meal. This bowl can now be used for anything to portion out a cup.

The same trick can be used for drinking glasses and beverages. The average glass in a cupboard is 8 oz.

**8 oz = 1 cup**

*What about foods where the serving size is in pieces?*

Pepper Jack Cheez-its

Serving Size: 25 crackers

Servings Per Container: 11

Calories: 150

One serving is 25 crackers, count out 25 on a plate or in our **cup** bowl to see what 25 cheez-its looks like on a plate or in a bowl. Do this until you get a feel for the portion size. Simply count out less crackers for less calories.

As our example we'll use peanut butter and cheez-its.

Bread - 40 calories per slice - 4 slices 160 calories

Peanut butter - 190 calories per 2 tablespoons - 4 tablespoons 380 calories

Cheez-its - 150 calories per serving - 1 serving

Total: 690 calories

**Accurately counting the calories on a plate is the first step toward a healthy lifestyle.**

A lazy person could use a knife to scoop out the peanut butter and lick it clean. They might pour out a pile of cheez-its based on their hunger. Let's say conservatively you use 6 tablespoons of peanut butter instead of 4 and 1.5 servings of cheezits. Suddenly the calorie count jumps to 955 instead of 690. That's a 38% increase in calories. Apply that to entering daily calories. Imagine entering 2200 calories when the actual calorie count was 3036. How could anyone lose weight using these methods of measurement? It is easy to see why so many people are overweight. People literally do not know how many calories they are consuming.

**Knowing how many calories are in a serving and accurately measuring out that serving are the keys to weight loss and maintenance.**

**Everything consumed in a day goes toward the total calorie count for that day - even cough drops and gum have a calorie count.**

*How will I know the serving size for a piece of meat?* Generally speaking, 3 oz of meat, fish, or poultry is equivalent to a deck of playing cards on the palm of your hand. For example, 3 oz of ground beef is 232 calories.

If you know the total weight of the package then you can divide out the portions based on the total calories for the package. For a 1 lb package of ground beef, do the math. 232 / 3 = 77 calories per oz. Depending on how it will be used, the ground beef calories can be easily computed. 1 lb of ground beef is approximately 1234 calories. If half was used in a casserole, that would be 617 calories. If four hamburger patties are grilled, each burger would be 308 calories.

***How will I know the calories for dishes that contain multiple items?*** Any dish, whether it's scrambled eggs, chicken casserole, or mac and cheese with tuna can be summarized by the total calories that go into the pan. Simply add up all the ingredients. This total is divided by the number of servings the dish provides. **Create a Calorie Label** for every recipe. If the chicken casserole has 3500 calories and the glass dish can be divided into 6 portions then do the math. 3500 / 6 = 583. Each serving is 583 calories. This can be easily accomplished using the **Saved Meals** function in the Fat Secret App.

# What's in the Calories?

Basically, food can be divided into protein, carbohydrates (sugars) and fat. While many "diets" want to eliminate one or more of these elements, the best approach is to eat foods that strike a balance between all three elements.

# Protein [3]

1 gram = 4 calories

Protein can be found in almost every part of the human body. The enzymes that drive chemical reactions and the hemoglobin that transports oxygen are composed of protein.

Amino acids are the building blocks of protein. They are created from the ground up or by changing other amino acids. The **essential amino acids** can only come from the food we consume.

Protein that comes from animals provides all the essential amino acids we require. There are other sources of protein like fruits and vegetables, nuts, grains and seeds, but they do not contain one or more of the essential amino acids.

The right amount of daily protein is necessary to insure robust energy, stable blood sugar levels, proper digestion, maintaining or adding muscle mass, and even helping our moods to be even keeled. Protein takes longer to digest burning more calories and allow us to feel full longer aiding in weight loss and maintenance.

The recommended daily allowance in the US for **women** is **46 grams per day** and **56 grams per day** for **men**. Finding your own balance and personal RDA for your body is key in feeling happy and healthy every day.

Foods are always composed of many things. Something high in protein is not simply composed of just protein. It may be high in fat content or contain excess salt.

Peanut butter is a good source of protein. There are 7 grams of protein in a single two tablespoon serving. There are also 16 grams of fat that account for 140 of the 190 calories per serving.

Steak is a wonderful source of protein. A 4 oz rib eye steak has 22 grams of protein but 20 grams of fat. The fat accounts for 180 of the 280 calories.

Canned tuna in water can be used in a multitude of dishes. A 5 oz can of tuna has 36 grams of protein and only 1 gram of fat. 155 protein calories compared to only 10 calories from fat.

A 3 oz serving of ham steak has 15 grams of protein and only 4.5 grams of fat but, the sodium level is 1000 milligrams of the **2300 milligrams that is recommended per day**.

A 4 oz serving of salmon has 24.5 grams of protein, 6.7 grams of fat and is naturally low in sodium.

It comes down to choices and balance each day, week, and month. Here is a basic list of good sources of protein: lean beef, pork tenderloin, seafood, white-meat poultry, milk, cheese, dairy, eggs, beans, and soy.

Reading labels will help you think about how many grams of protein you are consuming versus fat and sodium in any food. The Fat Secret App will breakdown all daily calories into protein, fats, and carbohydrates, as well as showing the RDA for each.

The bottom line is trying to consume healthy foods that fall within your daily calorie goal.

# Carbohydrate 4

1 gram = 4 calories

The body obtains energy from three sources: carbohydrates, fat, and protein. These sources are called **Macro nutrients** and the body needs large quantities of all three. They must be obtained through the foods eaten daily.

Carbohydrates can be broken down into the sugars, starches, and fibers, that make up dairy products, fruits and vegetables, and grain products.

The RDA for an adult is 135g. Each individual needs a personal objective based on the **Daily Calorie Goal**, weight loss or maintenance aim, their **Kryptonite**, and personal tastes. Carbohydrates should comprise 45-65% of total daily calories.

Carbohydrates provide the fuel for muscles and the central nervous system. They enable fat to be metabolized for energy instead of protein. The RDA is based on the carbohydrates needed for the brain to function properly. Depending on the type of carbohydrate, they can be a quick source of energy and affect our state of mind.

There are simple and complex carbohydrates. Simple carbohydrates contain one or two sugars, digest faster, and are absorbed quicker into the bloodstream. Refined sugar, dairy products and fruit contain simple carbohydrates.

Some simple carbohydrate foods contain **Empty Calories** like syrup, soda, or candy.

Complex carbohydrates that contain three or more sugars include: cereals, whole grain bread, pasta, beans, peas, potatoes, peanuts, corn and assorted starchy vegetables. They provide a steady supply of energy versus the surge of energy some simple carbohydrates cause.

Whole grains and vegetables are an excellent source of complex carbohydrates. They allow the body to store glycogen in the body for energy use versus breaking down protein. Protein is used in muscle and body maintenance. Too much glycogen is stored as fat.

The fiber found in complex carbohydrates reduces the risk of diabetes, coronary heart disease, and is essential for digestion and healthy bowel movements. The Institute of Medicine recommends 14g of fiber per 1000 calories.

High calorie carbohydrates that could be considered **Bad**: soda, pastries, white bread, white flour foods, and highly processed foods. Some of these are **Empty Calorie** foods and contain little nutritional value.

Lower calorie carbohydrates that could be considered **Good**: whole grains, fruits and vegetables.

**Good Carbohydrates:**

Low in - calorie, sodium, saturated fat, cholesterol, and trans fat.

High in - nutrients and fiber.

No refined sugar or grains.

**Bad Carbohydrates:**

High in: calories, refined grains, sodium, saturated fat, cholesterol, and trans fat.

Full of refined sugar.

**Benefits of Eating Healthy Carbohydrates:**

Good Mental Health, Excellent Memory, Weight loss, Weight Maintenance, Fine Nutrient Source, and Healthy Heart.

Any diet based on ***cutting out carbohydrates specifically*** can lead to health issues: lack of energy, dizziness, mental and physical weakness, digestive problems, constipation, and issues with the kidneys and urination.

Eating carbohydrates comes down to choices based on calories, type and amount of sugars, amount of fat, and whether they are simple or complex. Balance the desire for taste with healthy selections.

# Fat [5]

1 gram fat = 9 calories

Just like the other two macro nutrients, the right type of fat is a necessary part of any healthy eating regimen. Fat keeps us warm, promotes cell growth, and increases the absorption of fat soluble vitamins like A, D, E, and K.

There are **saturated** (solid like butter) and **unsaturated** fat (liquid like vegetable oil). A healthy eating regimen consists of less than 10% from saturated fat. Milk, cheese, and meat can contain saturated fat. Fish and poultry contain less saturated fat than red meat.

Saturated fat food items include: anything cooked with shortening, margarine, or butter; coffee creamers, whipped toppings, palm oil, coconut oil, snack items and desserts.

Another type of saturated fat is **trans fat**. This is a fat that has been changed through **hydrogenation**. It increases the shelf life of products making crispier crackers, and flakier crusts. Trans fat can be found in processed foods, crackers, cookies, margarine, and some salad dressings. The less trans fats eaten daily the better.

Eating **too much saturated fat** can **increase** the bodies levels of **bad cholesterol** and **increase** the chance of **heart disease**.

**Eating unsaturated fats** can **lower** the **bad LDL cholesterol** in the body. Unsaturated fats can be divided into monounsaturated and polyunsaturated.

**Monounsaturated fat** food items: canola, olive, and peanut oils; avocado and nuts.

**Polyunsaturated fat** food items: safflower, sunflower, sesame, soybean, and corn oils; seafood like fatty fish, shellfish, salmon, sardines, mackerel, and trout.

**Omega-3 fatty acids** (seafood) and **Omega-6 fatty** (liquid vegetable oils) acids are the two types of polyunsaturated fats.

Review the saturated fat, trans fat, total calories from fat, and the percentage of saturated fat in the daily calorie total before adding any food to the weekly plan or daily calories.

# Download Fat Secret App

The next step is downloading a tool that can do most of the math and work it takes to compute daily calories. There are many apps to choose from but, I prefer the Fat Secret App. This is the first and most important tool.

This app will look up almost any food or product as well as the menus of most restaurants and fast food establishments.

Create a login to access account information from any device or computer.

Click on your account designated by email to select settings. Under settings select RDI. Complete the information on this page and select calculate. The recommended RDI will be displayed and can be changed to a specific daily calorie goal.

Select home to go to the main information page. This page will show: calories remaining for the day, calories consumed, calories burned, and current weight.

Daily calories are now ready to be input. Selecting add food will open the food diary.

The day is divided into meals: breakfast, lunch, dinner, and snacks.

Clicking a mealtime opens the selection page where you can: **Search** for a food by title, go to **Quick Pick** and select foods by category and specific name, search **Restaurants and Chains**, search **Popular Brands** and **Supermarket Brands**. Using a cell phone there will be an option to **Scan the Barcode** of the product by selecting the barcode symbol in the right hand corner. This will pull up the product information if it is in database.

As an example we will use the *Broiled Salmon* eaten for lunch. Typing salmon into search brings up our selection: *Baked or Broiled Salmon* 4 oz boneless raw (yield after cooking) 157 calories.

Once selected the *Broiled Salmon* now appears under the calories for lunch. By clicking on this selection under the lunch calories all the nutritional information for this food appears. Editing this entry is also available.

***The serving size, meal, and description can all be changed or the entry can be deleted.***

*Broiled Salmon* will also appear under **Recently Eaten**. This and the **Most Eaten** category allow the selection of specific food entries eaten on a regular basis without having to look them up and edit each time an entry is made.

**Saved Meal** allows multiple items to be saved together as a meal. This saves time and effort for meals that contain the same food combinations each time they are prepared.

Scroll to the bottom of your food diary page to find a summary that includes totals for: fat, cholesterol, sodium, total carbohydrates broken down into dietary fiber and sugars, and protein. There is also a pie chart representing the percentage of protein, carbohydrate, and fat consumed.

Clicking on **reports** will show a breakdown in three different categories. The food eaten is broken down by calories, macros, and nutrients. Depending on body type, health issues, and types of foods consumed, you can monitor individual macros or specific nutrients. Under macros, the protein, carbohydrate, and fat consumed is displayed as a percentage of the total. Under nutrients, the macros are broken down by type as well as listing totals for cholesterol, sodium, and potassium.

Under **calories burned,** on the home page daily activities can be added as exercise. The app assigns 8 hours for sleep and 16 for rest. Any added exercise activities are subtracted from the 16 hours of rest. The calories calculated for sleep and rest are an approximation and may be higher than what your individual body burns. This, also, applies to the daily exercise activities. The number of hours slept can be edited each day.

Under **current weight** enter your starting weight and goal weight. This will track weight loss and show how many pounds to achieve your goal weight.

In the **Community** section, share your experience with others and draw support. Create a personal file of instructions and ingredients under **Recipes**. Share your daily calorie, nutrition, and exercise data with doctors, trainers, or councilors in **My Professionals.**

# Purchase A Digital Scale

The second most important tool will be a quality digital scale. A digital scale should give a consistent and accurate reading every time.

Decide what time of day and how often you will weigh. Morning can be a good time to get on the scale. Weigh before eating or drinking anything, but after going to the restroom. The number from the first weigh in is a **baseline**. Weighing on your **baseline scale** gives the most consistent results since other scales may have different calibrations. Depending on the time of day, food and drink consumed, digestion, and physical activity body weight can vary several pounds per day. Due to this variance weighing more than once a week could be detrimental to keeping a positive attitude about eating healthy and exercising if body weight swings up or down.

## Average Daily Calorie Consumption

Getting started week 1 is easy. Weigh and input that number into the Fat Secret App. The goal is to begin on a normal week without holidays, celebrations, or vacation time. Go thru a normal routine each day. If a normal week entails eating out for lunch 2-3 times, dinner twice, drinks 2-3 times, and grabbing a pizza to watch the game, then follow this regular pattern. Enter each and every calorie using product labels, correct portions, servings, and the Fat Secret App. Do not leave anything out or fudge any of the numbers, servings or portions.

Beginning week 2 look at the diet calendar under menu on the Fat Secret App. Scroll to the bottom of the page and you will see your average daily calories thru 7 days. Get on the scale to see if your weight has fluctuated more than 1 or 2 pounds. If your weight is within 1 to 2 pounds then the average daily calories thru 7 days can be a **baseline** for **A**verage **D**aily **C**alorie **C**onsumption. The baseline **ADCC** could be 2500.

# 4 Motivation / Obstacles

Why are you eating? / What time of day are you hungry?

What's your kryptonite? / What's your yearly cycle?

As our example, John's ADCC is 2500. Week 2 goal is going to be a 500 calorie per day reduction. In the Fat Secret App 2000 calories will be entered under RDI.

Before learning how to cut calories and eat the same foods, the motivation for eating and the obstacles to reducing daily calories must be examined.

## Why are you eating?

The obvious answer would be: because I am hungry. The reality can be a multitude of factors having little to do with actual hunger. Going out to lunch and eating a satisfying meal may be a way to get thru the day. That high calorie snack reduces the level of boredom. A big bowl of ice cream may ease the loneliness of watching TV alone. It's hard to attend a party or celebration and refrain from eating or drinking. Social interaction almost always involves some form of food or drink.

The key will be to ask yourself a simple question: Am I hungry? How hungry do I feel? What will satisfy my body and not my mental or emotional needs?

Actually being hungry will be sign you are on the right path. Balancing hunger versus mental or emotional needs will be the key.

***Eating alone is much liking drinking alone. It is a recipe for disaster.*** Eating with others during mealtime and for social interaction will meet mental and emotional needs.

Do you eat to feed your body? Do you eat to satisfy emotional or mental needs? There must be a balance to *Live Your Life, Forget the Diet, Find Your Zen.*

# The Daily Quotient

Daily Calories / Priorities = Balance

Each day pick one **eating event** that will be the priority for that day. Maybe Thursday is Xtapa Day at work. Everyone goes Mexican for lunch. This is Thursday's **eating event**. Plan ahead and enter the calories that will be eaten during Thursday's lunch hour the night before. This will leave X amount of calories for breakfast, dinner, and snacks. Inputting the calories ahead of time allows for being mentally prepared to eat less calories for breakfast and dinner. Deciding ahead of time what will be ordered and how many calories will be allotted will make eating out that much more satisfying. If additional calories need to be added, that's fine. Having a guideline can only lead to success.

Preplanning will work for almost any eating event. While the exact food or drink consumed may differ slightly, it can be estimated using the Fat Secret App. Whether it's beer, chocolate birthday cake, grilled burgers, potato salad, margaritas, cookies, or chicken casserole, counting the calories is easy.

If the eating event is spur of the moment, simply use the Fat Secret App to calculate what calories there are to work with to meet the goal for that day.

# What time of day are you hungry?

They say breakfast is the most important meal of the day but, if you consume all your calories then what will you eat the rest of the day? *Breakfast moderation is an important start to the day.*

33

Activia Light Yogurt has 60 calories and will start the day with probiotics. Probiotics are good bacteria that keep your digestive system healthy by controlling the growth of harmful bacteria. Making this part of my morning regimen has lead to a marked improvement in chronic IBS symptoms.

Here are the benefits of starting every day with a 100 calorie banana: source of key nutrients like potassium, moderate blood sugar levels, promote healthy digestion, aid in weight loss, contain powerful antioxidants, may lower appetite, and can reduce soreness and cramps from exercise. [6]

That's 160 calories and counting to start the day. Depending on hunger level and schedule more calories may need to be consumed to have a successful day. A glass of orange juice and a bowl of Basic Four with fat free milk adds 400 calories for a total of 560 calories.

Regardless of what time of the day you are hungry **do not skip meals**. It may be tempting to allot the calories to a certain time of day or a high calorie meal but your energy and blood sugar levels will suffer and so will your health and productivity.

Personally, my time is dinnertime. Eating anytime of the day is enjoyable but, I am always hungry at dinnertime. A balance must be struck between what is eaten for breakfast, lunch and snacks to allow enough calories for a satisfying evening meal.

Maybe dinnertime is not the time of day your body is hungriest. Maybe it is breakfast, lunch or somewhere in between. Finding the meal that brings the most enjoyment is key to planning a successful day.

The Fat Secret App shows at any point in the day the calories remaining based on what has been input. This allows for preplanning meals based on the allotted calories that are left for the day

.

# When is dinnertime?

Dinnertime is relative to work, family, traffic, appointments, errands, and preparation. Eating too late in the day can be undesirable for a couple of reasons. The later in the day dinner is eaten the more likely your body will be sedentary after eating the meal. Evening exercise can aid in alleviating this problem, especially if it is an intense workout that leaves the body in state of **EPOC**. The body digesting a large late night meal may affect the ability to get a good night's sleep. Generally speaking, eating dinner before 7 PM is a good rule of thumb.

Snacking is separate from dinnertime but, the calories count the same. If snacking during the evening while watching TV is a priority, then enough calories need to be left after dinner to stay within the daily calorie goal.

# What's your kryptonite?

**Two types of kryptonite:** What food or drink will absolutely cause a body to gain weight? What food or drink can a person not resist?

**My kryptonite** is *ice cream* and *peanut butter*. Regardless of daily calories or exercise if a bowl of ice cream is eaten several times a week, weight gain will be seen. Ice cream is indulged in only 6 times a year and not to be found in the freezer as a temptation.

Peanut butter on the other hand does not affect my body anymore than anything else that is 190 calories per serving. The problem is having it in the pantry. If the temptation is there, I will eat it on bread, crackers, a sandwich, or straight out of the jar daily. The fact that just two tablespoons are so high in calorie and fat makes it a difficult food to eat every single day. Peanut butter is only eaten at mom's house and never found in my pantry.

*It is important to note that ice cream and peanut butter have not been eliminated from Living My Daily Life, only moderated.*

Each individual will have to determine what foods fall under the two types of kryptonite for their body. Moderating and removing these obstacles will allow you to be successful to *Live Your Life, Forget the Diet, Find Your Zen.*

# Slow Down

The world runs at a fast daily pace. How quickly we eat meals and snacks is determined by stress, work schedule, time limitations, and a variety of factors. Two things happen when we eat at too rapid a pace: The satisfaction of flavor is lost and the brain does not have time to send a signal that we are full.

What's on the plate does not need to be finished if there is a physical sensation of being full. This allows for gauging future portions and eliminating extra calories.

# Determine Your Yearly Cycle

Every person that has struggled to maintain a goal weight has a yearly cycle. The cycle contains one or more periods where maintaining a goal weight is difficult or impossible.

Maybe during the winter months, when daily exercise is a challenge and cabin fever leads to boredom, eating becomes a daily focus. Shift the focus, get active and eat healthy.

Laying by the pool or lake and drinking beer in the summer seems harmless enough. Harmless if swimming and water sports help burn the extra beer calories.

Then, there are the holidays starting with Halloween, an entire day dedicated to eating candy. Thanksgiving, Christmas, and New Years round out a season of giving, thanks, and eating. Focus on a daily eating event, the daily quotient and meeting the weekly calorie goal. Find your Zen and keep at it thru the busy season.

My personal cycle begins with the start of football season. Each and every Saturday is always an excuse to eat and drink. This begins on Friday and extends thru Sunday. Traveling to away and postseason games only adds opportunities to try local cuisine and brews, special desserts, and sample the night life. It is a time to enjoy family, friends and fellow alumni. This coincides with the holiday season and could be called the perfect storm.

The normal year begins with cutting calories, exercise, and returning to a goal weight by summertime. Summertime is easy time. Easy to be active from sunup till sundown after 8 PM. Happy and healthy heading into a time of year when it is a struggle not to gain weight.

Knowing this a preemptive strike can be planned. Walking my dogs is my Zen. As football season approaches being on a daily walking regimen ensures calories will be burned and my metabolism will stay elevated. Choosing a **daily eating event** and maintaining the **daily quotient** are critical during this part of my **yearly cycle**.

Moderation and planning are the key to sustaining a goal weight during this part of the yearly cycle.

Determining and planning ahead for a yearly cycle will prevent backsliding and the need to cut calories to return to a goal weight.

Imagine not needing to lose the same 15-18 pounds every January 1st. Now that's how to *Live Your Life, Forget the Diet, Find Your Zen.*

# Vacation

Taking a break from the normal routine to travel and explore is a wonderful experience. Use common sense and planning when it comes to eating and drinking on vacation. The last thing anyone wants is a weight gain hangover upon returning home from a wonderful trip.

Take advantage of local cuisine and enjoy exotic food and drink but, set a **Vacation Daily Calorie Goal** intended to maintain the current weight.

When on holiday, the normal eating, sleeping, working routine will be suspended. Simply consider what the **Daily Quotient** will be each day using the **Vacation Daily Calorie Goal**, plan the **Eating / Drinking Event** each morning, consider the total change in mealtimes and adjust according to the days physical activities, be wary of your **Kryptonite**, and try to avoid **over** and **excess eating**.

Mentally prepare for the freedom to eat and drink throughout the day and set the Vacation Daily Calorie Goal. Take advantage of the local recreational activities and burn the extra calories consumed at the restaurant or bar. Make memories, return home refreshed, and best of all, return to a scale that reads the same number as when you left.

# Changing the Body's Set Point

Does the body have a set point and if so how can it be changed? Throughout a person's life based on age and physical activity, a person's weight probably hovers around a number until a change in lifestyle, activity, or age moves that set weight up or down. Maybe John weighed 165 in high school, 185 in the 20's, 200 in the 30's, and now finds at 45 his weight hovers between 262-268. Every year John loses 15 -18 pounds to drop down to 250. He would like to lose more but, his weight inches back up to 262-268 every year.

John finds his Zen and is more active walking dogs every day. Calories are counted and portioned properly so there is an accurate **ADCC**. The foods consumed are higher in protein and lower in fat with a balance of carbohydrates. The **daily calorie goal** is a 500 calorie reduction that equates to a loss of approximately 1 pound per week. The **daily quotient** is met and each day brings an **eating event**. John has determined the **yearly cycle** for his body and plans for the difficult time of year.

In a reasonable amount of time, John loses the normal 15-18 pounds and more. A goal weight is now conceivable and attainable. The slow weight loss means muscle mass was not sacrificed and the metabolism is actually higher.

This translates into John's set weight dropping to 250. It make take time to drop the set weight further and will take planning and motivation to maintain a goal weight but John will no longer be losing the same 15-18 pounds a year.

John has not starved or deprived himself. He is still able to enjoy eating and drinking in moderation. This is how to *Live Your Life, Forget the Diet, Find your Zen.*

# 5 Cutting Calories

Begin the journey by cutting 500 calories a day eating the same foods. John's ADCC is 2500 and he has a daily calorie goal of 2000. The key to *Live Your Life, Forget the Diet, Find your Zen* is eating foods that are lower in calorie or fat free.

## What makes food taste good?

Carbohydrates in sugar form, fat, and salt give the foods eaten daily the tastes we find appealing. Manufacturers actually aim for the right mix of fat, sugar, and salt to produce what is called the **Bliss Point**. The point where these three elements meet in perfect harmony to provide the right amount of sweetness, saltiness, and fullness of overall taste. The human body is programmed to seek out foods with these tastes. The response to eating these foods is a surge of endorphins that we will remember and seek out again and again. The right combination of these three elements is hard to resist. Learning to eat low calorie and reduced or fat free foods can reprogram the bodies desire for foods that provide us with an endorphin fix. [7]

## Soda

The elephant in the room is *Soda*. The average American probably consumes one or more regular sodas a day. A 12 oz coke can is 140 calories. A 20 oz bottle is 240 calories. If you drink two sodas a day the calories expended for soda range from 280-480. Potentially 25% of the daily calorie goal. In addition most sodas are caffeinated. Excess caffeine can cause negative health effects like digestion issues, nervousness, irritability, inability to sleep, headache and other chronic symptoms. [8]

The simple answer is diet soda. I limit myself to one caffeinated drink per day (12 oz diet coke). In addition many normally caffeinated drinks have a caffeine free diet version. Once converted to drinking diet, the taste of a regular soda will seem foreign and not taste as satisfying as the no or low calorie version.

Here is a short list of diet caffeine free drinks: **Diet Coke**, caffeine free diet **Dr. Pepper**, caffeine free diet **Mountain Dew**, caffeine free diet **Orange Fanta**, caffeine free diet **7UP**, caffeine free **Sprite Zero**, caffeine free diet **A&W Root Beer**, caffeine free 5 calorie **Minute Maid Lemonade**, caffeine free diet **Grapico**, and caffeine free diet **Twist**.

ADCC reduction from drinking a diet drink = 140 - 240 calories per day per soda.

# Everyday Foods

The easiest way to cut calories from the ADCC and eat the same foods is to consume the low calorie or fat free versions.

Many of the everyday foods found in the pantry can be replaced with low calorie or fat free versions with little difference in taste. Let's break down some of the common items found in the pantry where significant calories can be saved.

Sliced Bread = 70 calories per slice

*Low Calorie Sliced Bread = **40** calories per slice*

Mayonnaise = 100 calories per tablespoon

*Fat Free Mayonnaise = **10** calories per tablespoon*

Whole Milk = 160 calories per cup

*Fat Free Milk = **90** calories per cup*

Sliced American Cheese = 70 calories per slice

*Fat Free American Cheese = **30** calories per slice*

Cheez-its = 150 calories per 27 crackers

*Reduced Fat Cheezits = **130** calories per 29 crackers*

Wheat Thins = 140 calories per 16 crackers

*Reduced Fat Wheat Thins = **130** calories per 16 crackers*

Hot Dog Buns = 120 calories per bun

*Wheat Hot Dog Bun = **80** calories per bun*

Hamburger Buns = 150 calories per bun

*Wheat Hamburger Buns = **80** calories per bun*

Hot Dogs = 150 calories per link

*Fat Free Turkey Hot Dogs = **45** calories per link*

Margarine = 100 calories per tablespoon

*Light Margarine = **60** calories per tablespoon*

Beef Bologna = 90 calories per slice

*Light Beef Bologna = **60** calories per slice*

Yogurt = 100 calories per cup

*Fat Free Yogurt = **60** calories per cup*

Pudding Snack Cup = 90 calories

*Fat Free Pudding Snack Cup = **60** calories*

Cough Drops = 15 calories per drop

*Sugar Free Cough Drops = 5 calories per drop*

Chocolate Ice Cream = 287 calories per cup

*Fat Free Chocolate Ice Cream = 229 calories per cup*

*No Sugar Added Fat Free Chocolate Ice Cream = 180 calories per cup*

Ranch Salad Dressing = 140 calories per 2 tablespoons

*Fat Free Ranch Salad Dressing = 25 calories per 2 tablespoons*

Sour Cream & Onion Potato Chips = 150 calories per 15 chips

*Light Fat Free Sour Cream & Onion Potato Chips = 70 calories per 15 chips*

This is just a sample of the low calorie and low fat foods that can be substituted to reduce ADCC and eat same foods.

Looking for low calorie and fat free versions of foods can be challenging. Shopping at multiple stores is the answer to finding every low calorie or low fat food item on the shopping list. Stores may only keep a small quantity or a smaller size than is economical to purchase. Sometimes it is like a treasure hunt trying to find the low calorie and low fat items on the list.

Some of the calorie savings may seem small but, added up daily, weekly and yearly can make a big impact. Saving 10 calories every day for a year comes out to a savings of 3650 calories or 1 less pound gained.

70 calories a week saved = 1 extra pudding cup per week

Whether maintenance or weight loss is the goal, every calorie counts. **Calories saved are calories earned.** These earned calories give everyone the freedom to *Live Your Life, Forget the Diet, Find your Zen.*

# Calorie Comparison

As an example let's compare 1 Chili Cheese Coney Dog and Regular French Fries eaten at a fast food restaurant versus a low calorie low fat version prepared at home.

**Fast Food:**

Chili Cheese Coney Dog = 420 calories for 1 dog

Regular French Fries = 280 calories per serving

Medium 20 oz coke = 170 calories per drink

Total: **870 calories**

**Home Cooked:**

Fat Free Turkey Dog = 45 calories per dog

Wheat Bun = 80 calories per bun

Fat Free Cheese = 30 calories per slice

Fat Free Mayo = 20 calories per 2 tablespoons

Ketchup = 40 calories per 2 tablespoons

Mustard = 0 calories

Turkey Chili (no beans) = 24 calories per 2 tablespoons

Reduced Fat Cheez-its = 130 calories per 29 crackers or **equivalent**

Pickle Spears = 0 calories for 2 spears

20 oz Bottle Diet Coke = 0 calories

Total: **369 calories**

*Do the math: 870 - 369 = 501 calorie reduction*

That equates to a 58% reduction in calories for just one meal using low calorie low fat substitution while eating the same food.

*How can you compare cheezits to french fries?* Simply prepare some Ore-Ida Crispers Fries for the same calories as cheezits or chips.

Ore-Ida Crispers Fries = 230 calories per 20 pieces

Reduce the portion size to 12 pieces for an equivalent 138 calories

# Portion Size

Simply cut the portion size or quantity when low calorie and low fat are not an option. Eat the same food just eat less. Enjoy the **quality of taste** without having to have an **excess of quantity**. Use the daily quotient, daily eating event, and the Fat Secret App to meet the daily calorie goal while eating the same foods.

# Fast Food

In our modern fast paced society, fast food seems like a convenient economical way to simplify daily life. In actuality, the dollar menu is not your friend. Neither are the 4 or 5 dollar meal deals, coupons, afternoon specials, or discounts that entice overweight Americans every day.

The momentary satisfaction of eating a high calorie, high fat meal, connects with advertising to create a craving for something unhealthy.

A big mac and medium french fries is 870 calories, 91g carbohydrate (fiber 7g, sugar 9g 36 calories), 43g fat (saturated 12g 108 calories), 28g protein, and 1150mg sodium. The Fat Secret App will provide calorie information for most fast food establishments.

This equates to almost half of John's daily calorie goal. Taking into account a normal breakfast, John's calories at 12:30 PM stand at 1430 calories. 570 calories remain available to stay within the daily calorie goal.

Which type of **kryptonite** is a big mac and french fries? If it hinders weight loss, it may have to be moderated to once a month or less.

Will eating 870 fast food calories at lunch meet any of the bodies needs? Will it curb hunger and meet mental and emotional needs?

If making this a weekly **eating event** and planning to stay within the **daily calorie goal** will curb cravings and satisfy a personal need, then this is how to *Live Your Life, Forget the Diet, Find your Zen.*

A better way to meet the **daily quotient** would be to spend those calories eating and drinking healthier with friends and family.

The smart goal when starting a calorie cutting regimen in order to reach a goal weight is to **abstain from fast food for 3 months.**

Take time to eat alternate foods and change what the body craves. Garbage goes in, garbage comes out. The body will crave what it eats daily. Change what you eat daily and both mental and physical cravings will change.

Does that mean never eating a big mac and french fries? Remember, enjoy the **quality of taste** without having to have an **excess of quantity**. Limiting yourself to once a month will increase the satisfaction while lessening the unhealthy aspects of eating fast food daily or weekly

.

## Restaurants and Bars

The most important rule for eating out is to know the calories of what is being ordered. It is possible, but complicated, to estimate restaurant dishes based on the inability to know the types or quantities of ingredients used in preparation. Butter, lard, milk, cheese, and oil are just some of the high calorie ingredients that may be used in preparation.

The simple path is the Fat Secret App. If the restaurant menu items are not in the database, the business's website may include the calories for menu items. A server or manager may be able to provide a menu calorie chart.

John's eating event for the day is dinner and drinks at Chili's. The entire menu in is in the Fat Secret Database. Start by looking at the calories remaining to meet the daily goal. A moderate breakfast and dinner total 1100 calories leaving 900 for the evening meal.

**Appetizers** can be some of the highest calorie items on any menu.

Southwestern Egg Rolls = 810 calories for 3 rolls

Classic Nachos with Fajita Chicken = 1510 calories per serving

Spinach & Artichoke Dip with Tostada Chips = 1520 calories per skillet

Crispy Cheddar Bites = 1350 calories per serving

Calories can be estimated by dividing out the portions and being disciplined in the portion consumed.

**Reality Check:** Unless the appetizer will be divided among four or more people, it will be difficult to leave half or more of the dish uneaten.

**Entrees** offer many options that will fall with the eating event goal.

Margarita Grilled Chicken = 580 calories per serving

Chicken Enchilada Soup = 200 calories per cup

Santa Fe Chicken Wrap = 610 calories per wrap

Chicken Fajita Rice Bowl = 370 calories

Fajita Trio = 500 calories per skillet

Fajita Pita Beef Sandwich = 420 calories

Grilled Fish Tacos = 270 calories per taco

Half Rack Baby Back Ribs = 460 calories

Lunch Break Grilled Ham & Swiss Sandwich with Fries

 = 680 calories

6 oz Sirloin with Grilled Avocado = 410 calories

**Sides** offer an opportunity to add something healthy.

Sauteed Mushrooms, Onions & Bell Peppers = 160 calories

Steamed Broccoli = 40 calories

Spicy & Garlic Shrimp = 130 calories per 6 shrimp

Rice Pilaf = 105 calories

Caesar Salad = 260 calories

Rice and Kettle Black Beans = 290 calories

Mashed Potatoes with Black Pepper Gravy = 280 calories

Asparagus & Garlic Roasted Tomatoes = 70 calories

**Desserts:**

Sweet Shot Key Lime Pie = 240 calories per slice

Sweet Shot Red Velvet Cake = 250 calories per slice

Sweet Shot Warm Cinnamon Roll = 280 calories

**Drinks:**

Skinny Patron Margarita = 110 calories

Presidential Margarita = 291 calories

Strawberry Margarita = 387 calories

Tropical Sunrise Margarita = 174 calories

**Dinner & Drinks Eating Event 1:**

App - 1 Southwestern Egg roll = 270 calories

Entree - Cup Chicken Enchilada Soup = 200 calories

1 Fish Taco = 270 calories

Side - Rice Pilaf 105 = calories

Cocktail - Tropical Sunrise Margarita = 174 calories

Dessert - Sweet Shot Key Lime Pie = 240 calories per slice

Total: **1259 calories**

This example exceeds John's 900 calorie goal. If preplanning this **eating event,** cut 180 calories from breakfast and lunch in preparation of meeting the daily calorie goal. In the event dinner and drinks need to fall within the 900 calories remaining, simply eliminate one or more of the items selected for the meal. Skipping the egg roll appetizer puts the daily calorie goal over by only 99 calories.

Part of the journey will be to *Live Your Life, Forget the Diet, Find your Zen.* Coming within 99 calories accomplishes this while enjoying food, drink, atmosphere, and friends. The daily calorie goal is a guideline and should not become an obstacle to success.

**Dinner & Drinks Eating Event 2:**

This example will disregard meeting the daily calorie goal.

*App* - Spinach & Artichoke Dip with Tostada Chip

= 356 calories (1 of 4 servings)

*Entree* - Cajun Chicken Pasta = 1500 calories per serving

*Side* - Caesar Salad = 260 calories

*Cocktail* - Strawberry Margarita = 387 calories

*Dessert* - Molten Chocolate Cake & Vanilla Ice Cream

= 635 calories (1 of 2 servings)

*Total:* **3138 calories**

This is simply an **excess of quantity** in the form of calories. The **quality of taste** in both meals is equivalent. The difference being *1879 calories.*

# Alcohol

Drinking is part of the social fabric of American society. Planning and moderating the calories associated with this social interaction are critical. Start by selecting a designated driver, have a taxi service on speed dial, or Uber App on the cell phone.

***Drinking alone is as bad as eating alone. It is a recipe for disaster.*** Alcohol calories are **empty calories** but, mental and emotional needs can be met thru the social interaction it provides.

What's in the drink? What are the total calories? Is there a low calorie or diet version of the drink?

**Beware** of these pitfalls: oversized drinks, shots, and multiple liquor drinks.

**Beware** of the affect on the body: slows metabolism, dehydrates, and impairs judgement.

Impaired judgement may lead to a **late night fast food binge** on what become **deadweight calories.** These calories are nether needed or easily processed by the body in a sedentary state. It, also, wreaks havoc on the daily and weekly calorie goal.

When drinking beer, there are multiple options for going low calorie. Mixed drinks can use diet coke or other diet low calories options as the added component. *Do not skip dinner to meet the daily calorie goal.* It is important not to drink on an empty stomach. Try to drink water as the night progresses and drink water before going to bed. Limit mixed drinks using a caffeinated component. The mix of alcohol and caffeine can lead to severe dehydration and diarrhea.

Impaired judgement can cause the preplanning for a daily eating / drinking event to go out the window. It is important to know ahead of time the calories of the cocktails and how many will be enjoyed. The Fat Secret App should enable accurate calorie counting of any alcoholic beverage. In moderation, drinking can be part of a balanced healthy lifestyle.

Reality Check: When the planned evening has come to an end: *Go Home - Do Not Pass Go - Do Not Go to Another Club - Do Not Stop for Food.*

Think about this statement as a life lesson:

*Everything bad happens after 2 AM.* If you are out after 2 AM, take full responsibility for a lapse in judgement.

# Hydrate

The general rule of thumb is to drink 8 glasses of water a day. This may seem like a daunting task that hangs as a specter over every day. In reality many of the things consumed daily already contain water. A simple goal can be to alternate between a glass of water and other thirst quenching selections throughout the day.

Staying hydrated aids in weight loss, digestion, reduces fatigue, promotes healthy skin, and can relieve a hangover.

Add water to your day without feeling pressure to consume a certain quantity. *Live Your Life, Forget the Diet, Find Your Zen.*

# Sweet Tooth

A desire for confection after any meal may be referred to as having a **Sweet Tooth.** This is a craving that can be indulged with **quality of taste** instead of an **excess of quantity**. The taste of something sweet can be satisfying in a small portion.

Here are some examples of high calories sweets:

Hershey's Milk Chocolate Bar = 210 calories

Krispy Kreme Traditional Cake Doughnut = 230 calories

Krispy Kreme Lemon Filled Doughnut = 340 calories

Pound Cake = 350 calories for 1 piece (1/10 of cake)

Chocolate Cake with Chocolate Frosting = 235 calories (1/8 18 oz cake)

Cupcake with Frosting = 131 calories

Chocolate Chip Cookie (soft) = 69 calories

Peanut Butter Cookie = 72 calories

Chocolate Fudge = 90 calories per 1 cube inch piece

Blueberry Muffin = 313 calories

Fruit Danish Pastry = 263 calories

Apple Pie = 411 calories (⅛ of 9" dia)

Pecan Pie (Commercial) = 452 calories (⅙ of 8" pie)

Lemon Meringue Pie = 362 calories (⅛ 9" dia)

Ice Cream = 267 calories per cup

Peanut M&Ms = 250 calories per package

This is just an example of sweets with specific calorie counts. If the sweet tooth is indulged, know the exact calories being consumed. Desserts can be planned for and fall within the **daily calorie goal**. A specific confection may be the **eating event** of the day.

There are ways to indulge the sweet tooth in moderation. Low calorie and low fat versions of sweets are available. Eating a smaller piece or portion for **quality of taste** over **excess in quantity** is always an option.

Here are low calorie alternatives that provide the same taste of something sweet:

Jell-o Fat Free Pudding Cup = 60 calories (multiple flavors)

Hershey's Miniatures = 40 calories per mini candy bar (multiple types)

Reese's Puff Cereal (Dry) = 160 calories per cup

Activia Fat Free Yogurt = 60 calories

Kellogg's Cereal Bar = 120 calories

Cinnamon Toast Crunch Cereal (Dry) = 173 calories per cup

Strawberries 1 cup of halves / 4 tablespoons Redi Whip Whipped Cream = 109 calories

Peaches (Canned, Light Syrup) = 135 calories per 1 cup halves

These are just a few of my favorite go to low calorie foods that can be substituted for high calorie sweets. Any sweet dry cereal portioned out correctly makes a great snack. The mini candy bars can be broken up into 3 pieces to extend savoring each bite. It is possible to eat one cookie, doughnut, or piece of fudge. Enjoy the *moment of taste* rather then looking to over indulge in quantity.

When baking, use fat free or low calorie ingredients to lower the calories per serving. Bake in smaller quantities or sizes and share with neighbors and friends.

Indulging your sweet tooth thru planning and moderation is how to *Live Your Life, Forget the Diet, Find your Zen.*

# High Calorie Obstacles

Some foods are simply high in calories, fat, and carbohydrates. These foods may or may not be our kryptonite but can delay results on the scale or cause a backslide. These foods are satisfying on multiple levels and call to us in advertising, social settings and the grocery store.

**High Calorie Obstacle Foods:** Fast Food, Alcohol, Sweets, Peanut Butter, Pizza, Pasta, Ice Cream, Salad Dressing, Bread

Who doesn't love **Peanut Butter?** Eat it out of the jar, on a cracker, in a sandwich, or as a topping. High in protein but, high in fat and calories, peanut butter can only be eaten in moderation. 190 calories per 2 tablespoons is high calorie in low quantity. Taking a 3 month break from keeping it in the pantry can jumpstart meeting the daily calorie goal and reaching the first goal weight.

**Pizza**, need I say more? It is a go to food for the American family. Available in every size, shape, taste, cost, and preference, pizza can be baked at home, eaten in a restaurant, or delivered for convenience. Unfortunately, one slice of pizza is high in calories and fat.

Pappa John's Pepperoni Pizza = 340 calories per slice

Little Caesars Pepperoni Pizza = 280 calories per slice

Dominoes Pepperoni Pizza = 215 calories per slice

Pizza Hut = 230 calories per slice

Red Baron Pepperoni Pizza (Grocery Store)

= 185 calories per slice

Totinos Pepperoni Pizza (Grocery Store)

= 360 calories per half pizza

DiGiorno Pepperoni Pizza (Grocery Store)

= 200 calories per slice

It comes down to moderation, planning, and the daily eating event. Limiting a pizza meal to once a week or twice a month is a good start toward ensuring this will not be an obstacle to success.

**Pasta** is one of my favorite dishes. The variety of ways it can be served is endless and tempting. A small portion of any pasta will be high in carbohydrates and calories. This does not account for meat, sauce, butter, and other potentially high calorie ingredients found in the meal.

The key is eating a dish that has a balance of carbohydrates, fat, and protein for a reasonable amount of calories.

**Fettuccine** will be the first example:

1 cup cooked = 220 calories - 43g carbohydrates, 8g protein, 1g fat

Fettuccine Alfredo with Chicken **Milano's Grill**:

= **300** calories per cup - 28g carbohydrates, 19g protein, 13g fat

Fettuccine Alfredo with Chicken **Romano's Macaroni Grill**:

= **1370** calories per serving - 97g fat, 68g carbohydrates, 51g protein

The Milano's Grill Pasta Dish has a better balance of carbohydrates, protein and fat for the calories per cup. A 2 cup serving could easily fall within the daily calorie goal.

While tasty, the Macaroni Grill Pasta dish is top heavy in fat and calories taking up 68% of John's daily calorie goal.

**Spaghetti** as a home cooked meal and eaten at a favorite restaurant is the second example.

Spaghetti with Meat Sauce **Olive Garden (Lunch)**

= **710** calories - 94g carbs, 34g protein, 22g fat

**Home Cooked:**

Ronco Spaghetti = 210 calories per 2 oz serving (1 servings)

Ragu Light Spaghetti Sauce = 60 calories per ½ cup (2 servings)

80% Lean Ground Beef = 213 calories per 3 oz serving (½ serving)

Total: **436** calories 51g carbohydrates, 23g protein, 20g fat

*In the right balance, pasta can be a wonderful part of meeting a daily calorie goal that provides energy and taste satisfaction.*

Howard Johnson, Billy Moll, and Robert King wrote,"I scream, we scream, we all scream for **Ice Cream**". Few things evoke a sense of anticipation and joy like ice cream. An ambrosia for the senses it comes in any flavor, texture, combination, hard, soft, on a cone, in a dish, as a shake, or even a cake. The eating of ice cream may be a tradition enjoyed with family and friends. The social interaction can be priceless for creating lasting memories.

Ice Cream is normally high in sugar and calories:

Vanilla Ice Cream = 145 calories per ½ cup 15g sugar

Chocolate Ice Cream = 143 calories per ½ cup 16g sugar

Wafer or Cake Ice Cream Cone = 17 calories

Sugar Cone (Keebler) = 50 calories

Cake Cone (Kroger) = 20 calories

Ice Cream Cake (Dairy Queen) = 240 calories 24g sugar

Chocolate Triple Thick Shake (McDonald's)

 = 580 calories per 16 oz serving 84g sugar

Ice Cream Sundae with Fudge Topping (Whipped Cream)

= 437 calories 35g sugar

Strawberry Ice Cream Sundae Crunch Bar (Blue Bunny)

= 170 calories 13g sugar

The key is **quality of taste** over an **excess of quantity**.

It comes down to moderation, planning, and the daily eating event. Limiting ice cream to once a week or twice a month is a good start toward ensuring this will not be an obstacle to success. There are low calorie, fat free, sugar free options available as well as choosing to eat a smaller size, serving, portion, or quantity.

***Always look for a lower calorie option.***

Fat Free No Sugar Vanilla Ice Cream ( Blue Bunny)

= 80 calories per ½ cup

Sweet Freedom No Sugar Chocolate Ice Cream ( Blue Bunny)

= 100 calories per ½ cup

**Regular Salad Dressing** calories and fat can nullify all the benefits of eating a healthy salad for lunch or dinner. Let's say a half cup of dressing is an average for a large salad eaten as the entree. The following are all Kraft products.

Italian Dressing = 50 calories per tablespoon **400** per ½ cup

Ranch Dressing = 80 calories per tablespoon **640** per ½ cup

Thousand Island Dressing

= 65 calories per tablespoon **520** per ½ cup

Blue Cheese Dressing = 60 calories per tablespoon **480** per ½ cup

Honey Mustard Dressing

=45 calories per tablespoon **360** per ½ cup

French Dressing = 60 calories per tablespoon **480** per ½ cup

**Less is more. Simply cut the portion or try these Kraft fat free versions:**

Fat Free Italian Dressing

= 25 calories per tablespoon **200** per ½ cup

Fat Free Ranch Dressing

= 30 calories per tablespoon **240** per ½ cup

Fat Free Thousand Island Dressing

= 25 calories per tablespoon **200** per ½ cup

Fat Free Blue Cheese Dressing

= 25 calories per tablespoon **200** per ½ cup

Fat Free Honey Mustard Dressing

= 25 calories per tablespoon **200** per ½ cup

Fat Free French Dressing

= 35 calories per tablespoon **280** per ½ cup

All of these fat free versions may not be available when eating at a restaurant. Ask what fat free or light version is available. The dressing calories for most restaurants and fast food establishments can be found on the Fat Secret App. Getting the salad as takeout allows for using any fat free version of salad dressing you choose at home.

Simply going fat free and watching the portion allows for a tasty salad that falls within the daily calorie goal.

**Bread** has always been a mainstay for humans on Planet Earth. The baking of bread in various forms goes back thousands of years.

It can be found in almost every meal of the day. Depending on the kind of bread, calories, and carbohydrates, this can be good or bad.

**Whole Grain Bread Benefits:** low fat, cholesterol free, 10-15% protein, fiber, vitamins, antioxidants, and minerals; defense from obesity, heart disease, diabetes, stroke, and forms of cancer. [9]

**Healthy Bread Shopping Tips:** 100% whole wheat flour listed as first ingredient, 2g fiber per slice, and less than 200 mg sodium per slice.

Let's look at some delicious, but **high calorie** bread choices:

White Dinner Roll = 100 calories 19g carbohydrate

Hawaiian Dinner Roll = 140 calories 26g carbohydrate

Homestyle Yeast Roll = 170 calories 31g carbohydrate

Cinnamon Roll = 190 calories 31g carbohydrate

The Original Texas Garlic Toast (New York)

= 160 calories 17g carbohydrate

Grand Homestyle Buttermilk Biscuit (Pillsbury)

= 170 calories 26g carbohydrate

Sausage Biscuit (McDonald's) = 430 calories 34g carbohydrate

Breadstick (Olive Garden ) = 140 calories 25g carbohydrate

Side Bread and Butter (Outback Steakhouse)

= 156 calories per serving 26g carbohydrate

White Sliced Bread (Bunny Bread) = 80 calories 16g carbohydrate

Sliced Multi Grain Bread = 110 calories 22g carbohydrate

Sliced Banana Nut Bread (Market Basket)

= 170 calories 25g carbohydrate

Hamburger Bun (Cub Foods) = 120 calories 23g carbohydrate

Hotdog Bun (Publix) = 110 calories = 21g carbohydrate

This is a small sample of the bread products that will be a temptation throughout the day. There are low calorie, low fat, low sugar versions available for many of these items.

Moderation and planning will be the key when regulating bread consumption. **Moderation** in the form of excluding bread from certain meals or eating a single or half portion to stay within the **Daily Calorie Goal**. Planning for a **Daily Eating Event** that will involve high calorie bread products. Determining what foods in this category might be your **Kryptonite** and limiting them will ensure success in reaching and maintaining a **Goal Weight**.

To smell bread baking is a visceral experience. To see bread will make the mouth water. To taste bread will bring a smile to any face. It is everywhere; part of almost any meal and found in a multitude of forms.

*Breaking bread can be a part of everyday life with moderation and planning.*

# Fruits and Vegetables

The Good Earth provides that which is healthiest. From the vine, stalk, bush, tree, or root fruits and vegetables can provide almost everything needed to live a happy healthy life. They are low in calories and fat but, high in fiber, minerals, and vitamins; providing an excellent path to feeling full and reaching and maintaining a goal weight.

The ability to eat fruits and vegetables depends only on keeping the pantry stocked weekly. **To eat healthy, shop healthy.** A large variety of fresh fruits and vegetables are available year round. Take advantage of seasonal produce and stock up while it is available.

Cooking and eating can be quite the adventure with just a little bit of effort. Branch out and try something new once a month. The American Heart Association recommends eating 4½ cups of fruits and vegetables a day for the average adult consuming 2000 calories. Take this as an opportunity to add them to every meal.

**Here are some fresh and canned fruit choices:**

Gala Apple = 72 calories

Red Delicious Apple = 72 calories

Banana = 100 calories

Blueberries = 1 cup 42 calories

Cantaloupe = 1 cup diced 53 calories

Date = 23 calories

Figs = 1 medium 37 calories

Grapefruit = ½ medium 41 calories

Grapes = 1 seedless 3 calories

Honeydew Melons = ½ cup 30 calories

Kiwifruit = 46 calories

Mandarin Oranges = 60 calories

Mango = 135 calories

Nectarines = 70 calories

Oranges = 62 calories

Peach = 38 calories

Lite Sliced Peaches (Del Monte) = 1 cup 120 calories

Pear = 96 calories

Sliced Pears (Del Monte) = 1 cup 100 calories

Pineapple = 1 cup diced 74 calories

Pineapple (Del Monte) = 2 slices 60 calories

Plum = 30 calories

Prune = 20 calories

Raisins = ¼ cup 120 calories

Raspberries = 1 cup 52 calories

Strawberries = 1 cup halves 49 calories

Watermelon = 1 wedge 80 calories

**Here are some fresh and canned vegetable choices:**

Artichoke = 84 calories

Asparagus = 27 calories

Baby Carrot = 4 calories

Baked Potato = medium 194 calories

Beets = 1 cup 58 calories

Broccoli = 31 calories

Brussels Sprouts = 1 cup 38 calories

Cabbage = 1 cup 21 calories

Carrot = 25 calories

Cauliflower = 1 cup 25 calories

Celery = 1 stalk 6 calories

Cherry Tomatoes = 1 cup 27 calories

Corn = 1 cup 132 calories

Whole Kernel Sweet Corn (Green Giant) = 1 cup 120 calories

Corn on the Cob = 77 calories

Cucumber = 1 cup 16 calories

Eggplant = 8 calories

Garlic = 4 calories

Jalapeno = 4 calories

Kale = 1 cup 34 calories

Leeks = 1 cup 54 calories

Lettuce = 1 cup 8 calories

Mashed Potatoes = 1 cup 210 calories

Mixed Vegetables = ⅔ cup 60 calories

Mushrooms = 1 cup 15 calories

Okra = 1 cup 31 calories

Olives = 10 small 42 calories

Onion = 1 cup 67 calories

Parsnip = 1 cup 100 calories

Peas = 1 cup 117 calories

Sweet Peas (Green Giant) = 1 cup 100 calories

Pepper = 1 medium 30 calories

Pickle = 5 calories

Red Potato = medium 153 calories

Pumpkin = 1 cup 30 calories

Radish = 1 cup 19 calories

Spinach = 1 cup 7 calories

Squash = 1 cup 18 calories

Succotash = 1 cup 177 calories

Sweet Potato = 112 calories

Tomato = medium 22 calories

Turnip = 1 cup 67 calories

Yam = 1 cup 177 calories

Zucchini = 1 cup 20 calories

**Beans** are considered by many as a meat alternative. They are, also, a member of the Vegetable Group.

**Here are some fresh and canned bean choices:**

Baked Beans (Bush's Best) = 1 cup 340 calories

Black Beans (Great Value) = 1 cup 220 calories

Chickpeas (Progresso) = 1 cup 200 calories

Cooked Green Beans = 1 cup fresh 77 calories

Green Beans (Green Giant) = 1 cup 40 calories

Kidney Beans (Canned) = 1 cup 210 calories

Lima Beans (Del Monte) = 1 cup 200 calories

Pinto Beans (Great Value) = 1 cup 180 calories

Refried Beans (Old El Paso) = 1 cup 220 calories

When looking at canned fruits and vegetables, consider the amount of sugar and sodium that has been added to the product. All fruit has some natural sugar in it. Watch the labels for sugars that have been added to the syrup or juice. Buy canned fruit in light syrup or fruit juice. Compare canned vegetables to see which brand has the least sodium.

***Plan ways to add fruits and vegetables to breakfast, lunch, dinner, and snacks.***

Purchase the one step apple slicer and corer by ***Prepara***. With one push create a perfectly sliced apple.

Add bananas, peaches, strawberries, blueberries, or the fruit of your choice to cereal or oatmeal. Include tomatoes, mushrooms, onion, or bell peppers in an omelette. Eat melon wedges or balls as a side dish to brighten morning fare.

Carry a banana, orange, raisins, grapes, or an apple for that mid morning snack. The portability of fruit makes it a wonderful fresh treat anytime anywhere.

Choose a vegetable, salad, or fresh fruit as a side selection when eating at a restaurant or ordering takeout.

Select microwave meals that contain a healthy vegetable portion or add a canned vegetable or fruit to leftovers eaten during lunch hour.

Tomatoes can be added to many meals to add a vegetable serving: macaroni and cheese, scrambled eggs, omelettes, sandwiches, spaghetti, lasagna, salads, grilled skewers, or stuffed.

Sauteed onions, bell peppers, and mushrooms can be added to any dish that includes ground beef.

Create colorful tasty skewers for the grill that include: red bell peppers, onions, green bell peppers, tomatoes, yellow bell peppers, mushrooms, and squash. Put corn on the cob directly on the grill. Brush with BBQ sauce for added flavor.

Try a super salad with lettuce, tomato, cucumber, three types of bell pepper, squash, mushrooms, fat free cheese, croutons, chicken salad, and fat free dressing.

Add peaches, strawberries, pears, banana, or pineapple to jell-o.

Substitute chopped vegetables for chips when preparing a dip tray for celebrations, sporting events, or parties.

Substitute fruit for desserts by eating peaches, pears, or pineapple in light syrup. Lightly sprinkle strawberries with sugar and allow to set up in the refrigerator.

When sauteing vegetables, try to use healthier cooking oils: canola, corn, olive, peanut, soybean, and sunflower.

Try one new fruit and one new vegetable a month. The possibilities are endless for improving the taste and healthiness of each day's meals.

# Resetting Goals

Every day, week, and month there is an opportunity to reset the daily calorie goal. One day, week, or month does not define whether the current journey to a goal weight will be successful.

Start each morning with a clean slate. Work toward improving the ADCC for the week or month even if it has been a struggle. When a new week or month begins, put the results in the past and start fresh.

*Any progress is good progress.* Every pound lost puts the goal weight one week closer. Celebrate the victories, learn from the mistakes, and forget the failures of the past. Each and every day is an opportunity to move forward in all areas of life. Hitting the reset button applies to everything, not just weight loss.

# 6 Create a Meal Plan

Creating a plan for the meals that will be eaten in a given week should not be seen as a daunting task. When a plan is in place, it will actually simplify daily living and the weekly trip to the grocery store.

Once week one has been completed and the **ADCC** has been calculated, there is a daily calorie goal. Based on the **Daily Quotient**, **Eating Events**, the **Time of day you are hungry**, **Your Kryptonite**, and **Your Yearly Cycle** planning the week's meals is simply about choices.

Start by breaking the day into it's four components: breakfast, lunch, dinner, and snacks. For each component consider choices that will be satisfying and fall within the daily calorie goal. Break each component meal down into the individual items needed to prepare it.

**Breakfast Example:** banana, Activia Yogurt, Basic Four cereal with milk, and orange juice.

**List Items:**

Bunch Bananas

12 pack Light Activia Yogurt

1 box Basic Four

1 Gallon Fat Free Milk

1 Gallon Orange Juice

It is easy to substitute something in place of the bowl of cereal and banana: 2 scrambled eggs with tomato and cantaloupe.

**Additional List Items:** 1 dozen eggs, 3 tomatoes, 1 cantaloupe, light margarine.

**Lunch Example 1:** Lean Cuisine Chicken Fried Rice, Wheat Thins, Gala Apple.

**List Items:**

3 different Lean Cuisines

1 box Wheat Thins Reduced Fat

3 Gala Apples

**Lunch Example 2:** Two chicken salad sandwiches with tomato and mayonnaise, Cheez-Its, two pickles, and a diet coke.

**Additional List Items:**

1 container chicken salad

1 loaf Natures Own Light Wheat Bread

1 jar Kraft Fat Free Mayonnaise

1 jar Vlassic Dill Pickle Spears

1 12 pack Diet Coke

1 box Cheez-Its Reduced Fat Crackers

Once there are low calorie, low fat options in the pantry, food items can be mixed and matched to create a variety of meal choices.

**Dinner Example 1:** salad, chicken nuggets, french fries, pinto beans, strawberries / whipped cream

**List Items:**

2 lb bag Tyson Chicken Nuggets

1 bag Ore-Ida Krispers

2 cans Glory Pinto Beans

1 head lettuce

3 cucumbers

1 bag croutons

1 bottle fat free salad dressing

1 carton strawberries

1 can Fat Free Reddi-Wip

1 bottle ketchup


**Dinner Example 2:** pan-seared pork chop, sweet potato, great northern beans, dinner roll, and peaches.

### Additional List Items:

2 boneless lean pork chops

4 sweet potatoes

2 cans Glory Great Northern Beans

1 package small dinner rolls

2 cans Del Monte Light Peach Slices

1 bottle extra-virgin olive oil

1 bag flour

**Snack Options:** apples, yogurt, pudding cup, Wheat Thins, Cheez-Its, Hershey's Mini Candy Bars, canned peaches, strawberries, cereal bar, and dry cereal.

**List Items:**

1 box Kellogg Cereal Bars

2 boxes cereal

1 bag Hershey's Mini Candy Bars

1 package Jell-o Fat Free Pudding Cups

Using just these few examples a varied amount of low calorie, low fat food items have been added to the grocery list. Many of these items can be mixed and matched to provide variety in taste but uniformity in calories. There are multiple apps that will allow for the creation of a weekly shopping list but, a pen and pad is still a simple way to generate a checklist.

# Group Effort

Consider a partner, spouse, and family sharing the same household when planning weekly meals. Use this as an opportunity for everyone to participate in living a healthy lifestyle. It is never too early to include children in planning, shopping, and cooking the week's meals.

Separate family food items that fall into a **kryptonite** or **high calorie obstacle** category and store them in a different cabinet, drawer, or room.

You are never too young or too old to *Live Your Life, Forget the Diet, Find Your Zen.*

# 7 Planning / Cooking

Meal Choices / Recipes

**Anyone** can learn to cook. The best restaurant meal is easily replicated in your own kitchen.

Take the time to stock the kitchen with a basic array of pots, pans, utensils, measuring devices, handheld mixer, colander, cutting board, and tools for prepping fruits and vegetables. These items do not need to be expensive or unnecessary but, to succeed there is a right tool for every job. Over time the items that work best will find their way into your kitchen.

The **key** is to focus on one task at a time, use the proper pan, utensil, ingredient, temperature, and cooking time.

**Directions** are guidelines but, need to be followed to ensure the preparation is in the proper order. Once there is confidence in the ability to cook, be willing to alter directions and be creative with the meal that is being prepared. A slight alteration in ingredient, preparation, temperature, or time can make a big difference for better or worse in the outcome of the recipe.

The **first rule** my mother taught me when cooking was **clean as you go.** Put trash in the garbage, rinse and set used dishes or pots in the sink or dishwasher, return food items to the cabinet or refrigerator, and continually wipe the cooking area clean. Enjoy eating a wonderful meal without the worry of a piled up, messy kitchen waiting to be cleaned.

The **second rule** when preparing a meal is planning for the various dishes to be hot and ready at the same time. Utilize a strategy that uses the oven, stove top and microwave to ensure the entire meal is finished at the same time. Prepare items that take the shortest time and do them last. Cover pots, pans or plates with aluminum foil to keep items warm. If necessary meal plates (excluding bread) can be warmed in the microwave on high for

30 seconds to ensure everything is hot and ready. Bread can be warmed at 50% power for 10 sec per item.

# Google Search

**Food preparation** is a click away with Google. For example, search pan-seared steak and a multitude of videos and articles will appear. Utilize this vast array of opinions by experts to create your own method and recipe for cooking a pan-seared steak. This recipe will use the parts that suit your own personal tastes, judgement, and skill as a cook. Take notes that detail instructions and ingredients for all successful meals prepared.

# Family Cafe

Give the family kitchen a name: *John and Sarah's 3 Dog Cafe*. The name should be fun and represent everyone in the family. Create a **Family Cafe Menu** that lists favorite meals for breakfast, lunch and dinner. Include snack and dessert options as well as a *Fresh from the Grill* section. Continually update, add, change, and keep the menu current based on the time of year, likes and dislikes, and family consensus.

# Meal Cards

Use the notes from meals successfully prepared to create **Meal Cards** on index cards, apps on the phone and tablet, or a computer. The front of the index card should contain an interesting title, ingredients, and instructions for preparation. On the back, list grocery items and include total calories per meal or serving. Index cards can be kept in a box and organized alphabetically, by category, or mealtime.

**Meal Card Example:**

Side 1

Cassie's Colossal Chicken Casserole
cream potatoes, green beans, dinner roll

Ingredients and Preparation Instructions

Side 2

Grocery List

750 calories per plate

*Meal cards will speed up weekly menu planning and grocery check-list creation.*

# Calculate Calories and Macros for Any Recipe

Use the Fat Secret App as a recipe calculator. Go to any page of the daily food diary without entries . Enter the ingredients as food items.

Make sure the total amount of serving is entered under serving size. For example, a can of peas is 3.5 total servings if the entire can is used in cooking. The initial entry will default to 1 serving of ½ cup.

Once every item has been properly entered scroll to the bottom of the page to see the totals for calories, fat, cholesterol, sodium, carbohydrates (broken down into fiber and sugar), and protein.

Simply decide how many servings the dish will make and divide the totals by that number to create your own **Recipe Calorie Label**.

**To save this recipe:** click to add a food to any mealtime, select saved meal, click add new saved meal, enter recipe name, description, and select save. Select add food, check boxes of ingredients already entered for calculation and click check mark.

The meal info can be accessed, edited, or tailored for individual servings.

# Add Cinnamon [10]

Cinnamon can act like insulin which regulates blood sugar levels in the body. High blood sugar levels can cause an increase in the amount of fat that is stored making maintenance and weight loss difficult. Cinnamon aids in keeping unneeded fat from being stored.

Cinnamon directs an increase in metabolism that utilizes carbohydrates so they are broken down instead of being stored as excess fat.

The cinnamon itself takes longer to metabolize and this also increases the metabolic rate.

Cinnamon can lower LDL cholesterol, helps burn belly fat, and can suppress appetite.

Add to cereal, oatmeal, tea, coffee, cider, or fruit juice. Include in meal preparation and recipes. Purchase products that already contain cinnamon.

Consider taking a cinnamon supplement.

# Meal Plans and Recipes

The following meal plans and recipes come from my personal experience of learning to eat the same foods while cutting calories, bad fat, sugar, and portions. Cooking creatively for one person or multiple people is a learned skill that will serve for a lifetime.

Feel free to adjust these ideas and recipes to suit your personal tastes, cooking skills, and calorie goals.

# Breakfast

Breakfast is an important start to the day. Try to envision a meal plan that is creative and satisfying. Here are suggestions and recipes for the morning meal.

**Drink**: water, fruit juice, milk, diet soda, coffee, hot tea.

**Entree**: cereal with milk, Eggo Waffle, Pop Tart, scrambled eggs, omelette, fried or poached eggs, boiled eggs, oatmeal, french toast, fruit plate, or pancakes.

**Fruit**: banana, grapefruit, melon, grapes, strawberries, orange.

**Sides:** toast, cinnamon toast, biscuit, jelly/jam, light margarine, light syrup, microwave bacon, Fat Free Activia Yogurt, cereal bar, applesauce.

**Scrambled Egg Preparation:**

4 eggs and 4 tablespoons of light margarine

Beat eggs, melt margarine in non-stick skillet on low to medium heat, pour eggs into pan, salt as desired, continually stir eggs until they start to solidify, flip over until desired firmness. Add sliced tomato and pepper as desired.

As always, consider a portion that falls within the daily calorie goal.

1 scrambled egg with light margarine = 125 calories

**Omelette Preparation:**

4 eggs and 4 tablespoons of light margarine

Beat eggs, melt margarine in non-stick skillet on low to medium heat, pour eggs into pan, salt as desired.

Add: mushrooms, onion, bell pepper, fat free shredded cheese, leftover ham, turkey, chicken, or ground beef. Consider using a **Bird's Eye Frozen Vegetable or Medley Selection**. The possibilities are endless and totally based on personal taste. The vegetables and meat can be sauteed separately before being added. Either way, add the ingredients to the pan and let sit on medium heat for 2 minutes. As the mixture begins to thicken, lightly stir. Try to fold the eggs over as they firm up. The firmness and how well done the omelette comes out depends on personal preference. Add sliced tomato and pepper as desired.

### Sauteed Meat and Vegetable Preparation:

Enjoy chopping vegetables and preparing a plate for cooking. The more color and variety the better. Pour healthy oil into a non-stick pan set to medium heat. Once the oil is hot, add meat/vegetables and cook for 5-7 minutes (the time may vary, use your own judgement). Meat should sizzle when it hits the pan. Be careful not to get the pan too hot so the food is not seared. Stir occasionally and use a colander to drain when finished.

### Lean Cuisine Omelette Preparation:

There are many Lean Cuisine meals that can be used as the ingredients for an omelette. Simply follow the instructions for cooking in the microwave and then add to the pan of eggs and margarine.

**Lean Cuisine Omelette Options:** Shrimp and Angel Hair Pasta, Sweet and Spicy Korean Style Beef, Garlic Beef and Broccoli, Chicken, Spinach & Mushroom Panini, Chicken Fried Rice, Grilled Chicken Caesar, Cheese Lasagna & Chicken, and Ginger Beef Stir Fry.

There are a multitude of Lean Cuisine choices and they average around 300 calories per meal. This allows for quick preparation, cooking, and calorie estimation.

This is just one example of finding creative ways to cook low calorie meals that taste great.

Consider an omelette for lunch, dinner, or the family meal. The calories per serving are completely under your control based on number of eggs, tablespoons of margarine, and the added ingredients.

**Cinnamon Toast Preparation:**

There are two ways to prepare toast. Add margarine to a non-stick pan on low to medium heat and allow to melt. Add toast and coat bread allowing to brown. Margarine can also be spread onto the bread and then placed in a non-stick pan to brown. To spice up this morning meal lightly dust the buttered side of bread with cinnamon sugar and allow to brown as desired. The key to great toast is watch it cook and don't allow it to burn.

**French Toast Preparation:**

Ingredients: 2 eggs beaten, ¾ cup sugar, 1½ cups fat free milk, one cap vanilla, a sprinkle of nutmeg. Add cinnamon sugar to the mix or lightly sprinkle on during cooking.

Add the ingredients to a bowl one at a time and mix thoroughly. The amount of milk and sugar can be adjusted slightly after the first batch results.

The choice of bread is completely a personal choice but, white bread does seem to work better.

The mix makes approximately 10 pieces of French Toast and contains approximately 861 calories.

86 mix calories + 60 calorie white butter bread

## = 146 calories per slice

*Ways to reduce the calories per slice:* ¼ cup less sugar uses 19 less calories per slice, 40 calorie wheat bread uses 20 less calories per slice, less mix per slice will divide out to less per slice, 12 slices per batch reduces the calories by 14 calories per slice.

Using all three calorie cutting measures reduces the calories per slice to **93 calories.**

*Get creative with ingredients and portion size to cut calories while eating the same foods.*

### French Toast Cooking Instructions:

There are two options for pan depending on the type of French Toast desired: regular pan delivers a seared version closer to toast, non-stick pan creates a more dessert like pastry version.

For pan one dip each side lightly in mix and place in a pan on medium/high heat. For pan two immerse the bread on both sides and allow excess to run off before placing in a pan on medium heat. Flip to achieve even cooking until golden brown.

Lightly sprinkle cinnamon sugar halfway thru cooking to add a pop of flavor to the sweetness.

Use a thinner slice of bread for pan one and a thicker slice for pan two. Feel free to adjust the ingredients and cooking instructions to suit your own tastes.

**Pancake Mix Tips:** Follow the directions and use fat free and low calorie ingredients where available. The key is to be patient and allow the pancake to solidify before flipping the first time. Keep a watchful eye to see they do not burn.

**Microwave Bacon Tips:** Place bacon slices between two paper towels to absorb grease. Double the suggested heating time for crispy bacon.

# Lunch

The midday meal can be large or small depending on the day's activities, time, and calorie goal.

# Bake/Microwave and Go

**Lean Cuisine** is one of the best microwave lunch options. Here is a list of some of my favorites. The average meal is around 300 calories.

Marketplace Spinach Artichoke Ravioli

Culinary Collection Beef & Broccoli

Comfort Salisbury Steak with Macaroni & Cheese

Marketplace Spicy Beef & Bean Enchilada

Culinary Collection Steak Tips Portabello

Culinary Collection Salisbury Steak with Macaroni & Cheese

Market Collection Salisbury Steak

Simple Favorites Alfredo Pasta with Chicken & Broccoli

Simple Favorites Chicken Enchilada Suiza

Marketplace Sesame Chicken

Marketplace Sweet & Sour Chicken

Chicken Fettuccine

Marketplace Orange Chicken

Simple Favorites Lasagna with Meat Sauce

Cheese Lasagna & Chicken

**Season with salt and pepper.** Add a serving of Reduced Fat Cheez-Its or Reduced Fat Wheat Thins, an apple, or fat free pudding cup to complete the meal.

**Hungry-Man and Hungry-Man Select Dinners** are an excellent option when a stove is available. Be mindful of the calories and try to select an option under 600 calories. Eat a home cooked meal without cooking.

Here are some **Hungry-Man Dinners** that are less than 600 calories with a balance of fat, carbohydrate, and protein.

*Salisbury Steak with Mushroom and Onions*

Calories: 590 | Fat: 33g | Carbs: 52g | Protein: 22g

*Roasted Carved White Meat Turkey*

Calories: 420 | Fat: 10g | Carbs: 61g | Protein: 18g

*Country Fried Chicken*

Calories: 520 | Fat: 29g | Carbs: 51g | Protein: 18g

*Home-Style Meatloaf*

Calories: 530 | Fat: 22g | Carbs: 64g | Protein: 20g

*Grilled Beef Patty (slightly more than 600)*

Calories: 610 | Fat: 40g | Carbs: 38g | Protein: 21g

*Fiesta Beef Enchiladas With Rice and Beans*

Calories: 570 | Fat: 21g | Carbs: 83g | Protein: 18g

*Fajita Chicken*

Calories: 480 | Fat: 8g | Carbs: 79g | Protein: 30g

*Grilled Beef Patties*

Calories: 450 | Fat: 22g | Carbs: 39g | Protein: 24g |

Here are some **Hungry-Man Select Dinners** that are less than 600 calories with a balance of fat, carbohydrate, and protein.

*Slow-cooked Seasoned Pulled Pork*

Calories: 540 | Fat: 11g | Carbs: 73g | Protein: 29g

*Popcorn Chicken with Gravy Fries (slightly more than 600)*

Calories: 610 | Fat: 25g | Carbs: 62g | Protein: 27g

*Country Fried Steak*

Calories: 580 | Fat: 22g | Carbs: 77g | Protein: 1g

While some of these dinners are higher in fat than we might like, they offer a much better option than eating at Cracker Barrel, a real Mexican restaurant, or high calorie buffet. Take note of the sodium content and try to stay within the RDI of 2300 milligrams. The Grilled Beef Patties meal has 1160mg of sodium or 48% of RDI.

The calories easily fall with the daily calorie goal and with a little salt and pepper taste as good as a home cooked meal.

Knowing the exact calories makes for easy weekly planning.

**Campbell's Soups** are a hearty choice for lunch or dinner. Simply add Reduced Fat Club Crackers or Reduced Fat Ritz Crackers.

Heat 1 bowl of soup two minutes on high in a microwave.

Here are some examples of tasty Campbell's Chunky Soups:

There are **2 servings in one can** of Campbell's Chunky Soup. The calories below reflect the entire can.

*Chunky Fajita Beef* 320 Calories

*Chunky Savory Vegetable* 200 Calories

*Chunky Jazzy Jambalaya* 280 Calories

*Chunky Beef Burrito* 340 Calories

*Chunky Chicken Broccoli Cheese & Potato* 380 Calories

*Chunky New England Clam Chowder* 360 Calories

*Chunky Jammin' Jerk Chicken with Rice & Beans* 360 Calories

*Chunky Classic Chicken Noodle Soup* 220 Calories

Season with salt and pepper.

**Leftovers** make the best lunch meal because all the work except for warming in the microwave is done. Keep every small portion of evening meals and combine into lunch plates.

# As is, No Warming or Cooking Needed

**Sandwiches** are the *Undiscovered Country* of meals. Limitless variety, substance, texture, taste, and combinations provide an easy option for lunch or dinner.

*First, choose the bread.* Better to eat bread that satisfies your personal tastes than to get caught up eating the lowest calorie option. Try different low calorie, white, wheat, and multi grain options till one is found that strikes a balance between calories per slice and taste.

*Second, use Kraft Fat Free Mayonnaise.* 10 calories per tablespoon versus 100 for regular mayonnaise opens the door for creating a low calorie sandwich from normal ingredients.

*Third, use Fat Free Cheese.* 25-30 calories versus 120 for regular cheese allows the calories to be used elsewhere in the sandwich.

*Fourth, look for fat free*, light, or low calorie *lunch meats* like turkey, bologna, and ham.

*Fifth, keep lettuce and tomato* in the refrigerator to add a serving of vegetables to sandwiches. *Add Pepper* to sliced tomatoes to add a zing of flavor.

*Sixth, try Honey Mustard* Mustard instead of plain mustard to spice up any sandwich.

*Seventh, keep pickle spears on hand* for most sandwich meals to enliven the taste.

*Eighth, buy fat free or low calorie crackers and chips* to have as a side with sandwich meals.

*Ninth, consider toasting the bread* for certain sandwich choices.

**A Few Sandwich Options:** chicken salad, pimento salad, egg salad, tuna salad, StarKist Tuna Creations, ham, turkey, bologna, PB&J, banana, BLT, cheese, grilled cheese, BBQ, peanut butter, and scrambled egg.

*Using the guidelines presented here are some examples of tasty sandwich preparation:*

Add lettuce and peppered tomatoes to chicken salad, egg salad, ham, turkey, bologna, and scrambled egg sandwiches.

Use peanut butter on one side and mayonnaise on the other side of a banana sandwich.

Consider toasting the bread for chicken salad, BLT, and scrambled egg sandwiches.

Add Honey Mustard Mustard and cheese to ham, turkey or bologna sandwiches.

Consider adding a lunch meat like turkey and pickles to a grilled cheese sandwich.

Use more than one flavor of preserves when making two PB&J sandwiches.

Add pickles and coleslaw to BBQ sandwiches.

Pickles and Reduced Fat Cheez-Its or Reduced Fat Wheat Thins complete any sandwich meal.

As always look at the **Daily Calorie Goal** and the **Daily Quotient** to create a sandwich meal that fits your plan.

The average sandwich meal is around **500 calories** (excluding any that include peanut butter).

## Grilled Cheese Sandwich Preparation:

Add light margarine to a non-stick pan on low to medium heat and allow to melt. Add bread and coat allowing to brown. Margarine can also be spread onto the bread and then placed in a non-stick pan to brown. Place one piece of fat free cheese on each slice while buttered side browns so it can begin to melt. Add light turkey lunch meat and small pickles to one slice. Flip the cheese only slice on top to complete sandwich. Press down slightly and flip occasionally until golden brown and cheese has properly melted.

Add a bowl of Campbell's Tomato or Tomato Bisque Soup to spice up this meal. Use Fat Free Milk in place of water to create a thicker, creamier soup. Season with salt and pepper as desired.

**Cereal** or a **fruit plate** can be eaten at any meal especially lunch.

## Salad Preparation for Work Lunch:

Cut up lettuce, tomato, cucumber, squash, bell pepper, and strawberries the night before and place in reusable container. Carry Fat Free Salad Dressing, croutons, and chicken salad separately to add during mealtime. Include Reduced Fat Club or Ritz Crackers.

## Caesar Salad Kit:

There are multiple Caesar Salad Kit options in the produce section of any store. Choose the one that meets your personal taste and calorie goal. Add a tomato and cucumber to any kit.

## Wendy's Salads:

*BBQ Ranch Chicken Salad* 580 Calories

*Chicken Caesar Salad with Grilled Chicken Fillet* 340 Calories

*Power Mediterranean Chicken Salad* 340 Calories

Many fast food restaurants have excellent salad choices. Check the calories per salad and ask for fat free dressing.

**StarKist Tuna Creations:**

70-110 calorie pouches of premium tuna, select spices and ingredients can be added to a salad, sandwich, or eaten straight from the pack.

Hickory Smoked Tuna = 110 calories, 3.5g fat (0.5g saturated fat), 19g protein, 360mg sodium

Ranch Tuna = 80 calories, 2g fat (0.5g saturated fat), 1.5g carbohydrate, 14g protein, 360mg sodium

Sweet and Spicy Tuna = 90 calories, 0.5g fat, 4g carbohydrate (Sugar 3.5g), 16g protein, 380mg sodium

Hot Buffalo Style Tuna = 70 calories, 0.5g fat (0.5g saturated fat), 15g protein, 620mg sodium

Zesty Lemon Pepper Tuna = 80 calories, 0.5g fat, 18g protein, 290mg sodium

# Enjoy the Process of Cooking

Cooking dinner can and should be a fun experience. Enjoy the process of cooking any meal. Gather the family for conversation and inclusion in food preparation. Turn on some music, pour a glass of wine and savor the sights and smells of creating a family meal.

Set a great table for every family meal. The look of the table should be as appealing as the plate of food. Clear the room of clutter and unnecessary items. Make it a tech free zone and take a break from cell phones and tablets.

Use fresh and interesting items where possible for each meal. Create a colorful plate of chopped vegetables before making skewers or sauteing in a pan. Soak in the color and freshness of the **Good Earth.** Let the aroma fill the room and the house with anticipation. Include children in table setting, food preparation, and cooking.

Take the time to create an image with each plate of food that looks as good displayed as it tastes.

Give thanks as a group before partaking of the meal that in itself is a gift. Finish by clearing and cleaning as a group to efficiently leave the **Family Cafe** ready for the next meal.

# Dinner

The evening meal can be as simple or as complex as you desire. Many of the items discussed for breakfast or lunch will find their way onto the weekly dinner plan. Here are some meals and recipes to consider for dinner.

# Helper Meals

Betty Crocker **Helper** Meals (hamburger, chicken, tuna, Asian) offer easy preparation, variety, ability to reduce the calories per serving, and an option to spice up any meal by adding vegetables or exchanging one meat for another.

**Preparation:** Follow the simple instructions except for the amount of water and milk to be added. My personal preference and experience has shown better results by using 25-33% less liquid than the recipe instructs. If 2½ cups of milk and 1½ cups of water are required substitute 2 cups of milk and 1 cup of water. Use personal judgement and taste to determine if this suits your needs.

**Calorie Reduction:** Start by using fat free milk and light margarine. 56 calories less per cup of milk and 40 calories less per tablespoon of butter. Use a 12 oz can of *Chunk Light Tuna* in water versus a pound of chicken breast for a 170 calorie reduction. Consider no milk or margarine at all in the preparation. Use lean beef cooked in healthy oil for ground beef meals.

Simply look at the total calories for the entire dish and subtract the calories saved by using lower calorie ingredients or excluding an ingredient. This number can be divided by four, five, or six depending on the portion size that is desired.

**Add Vegetables and Swap Meats:** Add bell pepper and onion to any dish with ground beef. Feel free to swap tuna and chicken in any recipe. Add peas, carrots or both to any chicken or tuna meal. Consider using a **Bird's Eye Frozen Vegetable or Medley Selection**. Top hamburger, chicken, or tuna dishes with sliced tomato. Remember to season with salt and pepper.

Feel free to get creative with meat, vegetables, and spices when preparing any *Helper* meal.

Remember to accurately calculate the total calories in the dish and to portion out evenly based on the decided serving size whether it's four, five, or six.

Consider the label when choosing the right Helper meal to fit the weekly meal plan. Consider the calories per serving, daily calorie goal, and the balance of carbohydrate, fat, and protein in each serving.

Examples of *Tuna Helper Meals*:

Cheesy Pasta = 270 calories per cup

Creamy Broccoli = 260 calories per cup

Creamy Pasta = 250 calories per cup

Tetrazzini = 270 calories per cup

Examples of *Chicken Helper Meals:*

Fettuccine Alfredo = 310 calories per cup

Asian Helper - Chicken Fried Rice = 280 calories per cup

Cheesy Chicken Enchilada = 330 calories per cup

Creamy Chicken and Noodles = 280 calories per cup

Examples of *Hamburger Helper Meals:*

Stroganoff = 220 calories per cup

Philly Cheesesteak = 310 calories per cup

Lasagna = 280 calories per cup

Beef Fried Rice = 300 calories per cup

There are 40 meals to choose from so finding a selection that fits into the **Weekly Meal Plan** and **Daily Calorie Goal** should be easy.

Add a side salad, vegetable, and low calorie bread to expand any meal.

# Canned Vegetables

**Canned vegetables** are an easy way to add something healthy to every evening meal. My personal choice for canned vegetables is *Glory Canned Vegetables.*

Some Glory Products: pinto beans, great northern beans, green beans, green beans and potatoes, or red beans and rice.

If Glory Foods are not available in your area check out www.gloryfoods.com to order online and find recipes using their products.

Glory Pinto Beans: ½ cup = 130 calories, 1g fat, 18g carbohydrate(6g fiber, 2g sugar), 6g protein, 570mg sodium.

Glory Green Beans: ½ cup = 30 calories, 1g fat, 5g carbohydrate (2g fiber, 2g sugar),1g protein., 380mg sodium.

**Glory also offers low sodium options.**

Low Sodium Pinto Beans: ½ cup = 100 calories, 0.5g fat, 18g carbohydrate (6g fiber, 1g sugar), 6g protein, 250mg soduim.

**If daily sodium levels are exceeding the RDI look for the low sodium versions of the canned vegetable brands on the grocery list.**

**Del Monte Selections:** mixed vegetables and sweet peas.

Del Monte Mixed Vegetables: ½ cup = 45 calories, 0g fat, 9g carbohydrate (3g fiber, 3g sugar), 2g protein, 310mg sodium.

*Del Monte No Salt Added Mixed Vegetables:* ½ cup = 40 calories, 0g fat, 8g carbohydrate (2g fiber, 3g sugar), 2g protein, 25mg sodium.

Del Monte Sweet Peas: ½ cup = 60 calories, 0g fat, 13g carbohydrate (4g fiber, 6g sugar), 3g protein, 390mg sodium.

*Del Monte No Salt Added Sweet Peas:* ½ cup = 60 calories, 0g fat, 15g carbohydrate (4g fiber, 4g sugar), 4g protein, 10mg sodium.

Almost every vegetable is available canned. Take the time to locate stores that carry your favorite canned vegetable selection.

# Bake, Boil, Microwave

Many simple evening meals can be baked, boiled, or warmed in microwave with little effort.

**Sweet Sue Chicken and Dumplings with Sweet Peas:** Drain liquid from Sweet Sue Chicken and Dumplings and pour into microwave safe container (3 cups); drain can of no salt added sweet peas and pour ½ can into container (about 1 cup); heat for 3 minutes on high. Makes 2 servings as entree or 4 servings as a side dish.

Total calories = 675

entree serving = 338 calories, 7.5g fat (3g saturated), 45g carbohydrate (8g fiber), 23g protein

side dish serving = 169 calories


**Chicken, Shells and Cheese Preparation:**

½ package Ronco Large Sea Shells Pasta, 8 slices Fat Free Kraft or Borden Cheese, 8 tablespoons light margarine, 1 can sweet sue chunk chicken, 1 large tomato

Follow directions to prepare ½ package Ronco Large Sea Shells Pasta. Drain can of chicken. Using a 8x8 inch glass dish lay out four slices of cheese and four tablespoons of butter, heat in microwave for one minute on high. Pour in pasta shells and 1 can chicken, lay four slices of cheese and four tablespoons of butter on top, heat on high 3 minutes, and mix thoroughly. Heat 3-5 minutes on high and stir. Top with slice tomato and pepper. Makes 6-8 servings. Light Chunk Tuna in water can be substituted for chicken.

Total calories = 1800

6 serving entree = 300 calories per serving, 9g fat, 30g carbohydrate (1.25g fiber, 2.5g sugar), 21g protein

8 serving side = 225 calories per serving

## Chicken Nuggets and Fries Preparation:

Tyson Chicken Nuggets and Ore-Ida Crisper Fries

Preheat the oven to 425 degrees. Place desired number of nuggets and fries in a pan sprayed with *Pam*. Bake for 12-14 minutes turning nuggets and stirring fries at halfway point.

7 nuggets and 10 fries = 493 calories, 31g fat (8g saturated), 33g carbohydrate (2g fiber), 20g protein

For added kick if there are calories available use Kraft Honey BBQ Sauce as a dip at 30 calories per tablespoon. Ketchup is 20 calories per tablespoon.

Add a side salad, canned vegetable, sliced tomato, or fruit to complete the meal.

## Chili Cheese Dog Preparation:

Finding low calories hot dogs can be a challenge. The 60 calorie Oscar Meyer Lean Beef Hot Dogs are a good compromise. Kraft Fat Free Cheese (25 calories), wheat buns (80 calories), Hormel 98% Fat Free Turkey Chili No Beans 24 calories per 2 tablespoons, Kraft Fat Free Mayonnaise 10 calories per tablespoon, mustard (zero calories) and ketchup 20 calories per tablespoon.

Boil hotdogs. Warm chili in microwave. Spread mayonnaise on bun and lay one slice of cheese in middle. Warm bun in microwave on 50% power for 30 seconds or until cheese melts. Place hotdog in bun and top with mustard, ketchup, and chili.

1 chili cheese dog = 219 calories

Additional toppings: pickles, relish, coleslaw.

**Pizza recommendations:** Red Baron and Totinos Party Pizza produce the most satisfying results considering the low cost, quality of taste, and consistency with which they cook.

**Red Baron Classic Crust Pepperoni Pizza** = 370 calories per 2 slices, 17g fat (8g saturated), 41g carbohydrate (2g fiber, 8g sugar), 15g protein

Red Baron Classic Crust Supreme Pizza = 320 calories per 2 slices, 14g fat (7g saturated), 35g carbohydrate (2g fiber, 7g sugar), 13g protein

Red Baron Classic Crust Hamburger Pizza = 388 calories per 2 slices, 16g fat (8g saturated), 41g carbohydrate (2.5g fiber, 5g sugar), 19g protein

The **Totinos Party Pizzas** come in a rectangle and can be cut into various serving sizes.

Classic Pepperoni = 360 calories per half pizza, 19g fat (5g saturated), 36g carbohydrates (2g fiber, 4g sugar), 11g protein

Combination = 370 calories per half pizza, 20g fat (6g saturated), 36g carbohydrates (2g fiber, 4g sugar), 12g protein

Supreme = 350 calories per half pizza, 17g fat (4.5g saturated), 37g carbohydrates (2g fiber, 4g sugar), 12g protein

Hamburger = 370 calories per half pizza, 19g fat (4g saturated), 34g carbohydrates (2g fiber, 3g sugar), 16g protein

**Seafood Meal Recommendation:**

**Gorton's** makes a variety of seafood products that are easy to bake in the oven. There are many grilled low calorie options.

**Seafood Meal Example 1:** 1 Gorton's Crunchy Fish Stick, 5 Gorton's Jumbo Butterfly Shrimp, 2 hush puppies, and Ore-Ida Crispers Fries.

Seafood Plate = 530 calories

**Seafood Meal Example 2:** 2 Gorton's Grilled Tilapia Fillets, 8 Gorton's Classic Grilled Shrimp, 8 Gorton's Clam Strips, and Ore-Ida Steak Fries.

Seafood plate = 510 calories

*Include calories for sauces or condiments.*

Add a side salad, canned vegetable, and fruit to complete the meal.

**Aluminum Foil Chicken and Vegetable Preparation:**

1 Boneless skinless chicken breast, baby carrots, 1 medium squash, 1 half medium onion, 2 medium potatoes, 1 bag Bird's Eye Steamfresh Asian Medley Vegetables, 2 tablespoons light margarine, and aluminum foil.

Season chicken with tenderizer and let sit while doing prep work. Microwave Asian Medley Vegetables in bag. Cut up squash, onions, and potatoes. Boil potatoes and baby carrots 10 minutes. Melt 2 tablespoons light margarine per piece of chicken. Start with a 12x12 inch piece of foil and place 1 chicken breast in the center, cover with onion, and season with salt and pepper. Top with Asian Medley Vegetables, half of melted margarine, add squash, potatoes, baby carrots, and rest of margarine. Season with salt and pepper. Close up the foil and place in baking pan. Bake at 425 for about 1 hour.

Use pot holder to remove foil from pan and empty contents onto plate.

This is a simple but filling and satisfying meal. Feel Free to add additional vegetables of your choice. Consider using any **Bird's Eye Frozen Vegetable or Medley Selection.**

**Knorr** offers a wide range of pasta, rice, and fiesta side dishes prepared on the stovetop with little effort. The packages also include recipes for expanding the side to an entire meal.

*Fiesta Sides Spanish Rice* = 230 calories per cup prepared, 1g fat, 49g carbohydrate (fiber 2g, sugar 3g), protein 6g

**Here is an example of a Knorr Recipe for Fiesta Sides Spanish Rice:**

1 lb lean ground beef, 1 ⅔ cups water, 1 can whole kernel corn undrained, 1 package Fiesta Sides Spanish Rice, ¾ cup fat free cheddar shredded cheese

1. Brown meat in nonstick skillet, add water, bring to boil, add Spanish Rice, and bring to boil.

2. Reduce heat and simmer uncovered, stirring occasionally. 10 minutes or until rice is tender.

3. Stir in ½ cup cheese until melted; top with ¼ cup cheese.

Use Fat Secret to calculate the calories and nutritional information for this meal and add to saved meals. Decide on the number of portions and divide that number into the calorie and nutritional totals.

**Fiesta Sides Mexican Rice**= 280 calories per ½ cup prepared, 1g fat, 50g carbohydrate (fiber 2g, sugar 1g), 7g protein

**Asian Sides Chicken Fried Rice** = 290 calories per cup prepared, 1.5g fat, 48g carbohydrate (fiber 2g, sugar 2g), 7g protein *(Add Bird's Eye Steamfresh Stir Fry Vegetables)*

**Asian Sides Teriyaki Rice** = 280 calories per cup prepared, 1.5g fat, 49g carbohydrate (fiber 2g, sugar 4g), 5g protein *(Add Bird's Eye Steamfresh Teriyaki Stir Fry Vegetables)*

Consider adding a **Bird's Eye Frozen Vegetable or Medley Selection** to any of the Knorr Fiesta Sides.

Read the labels to choose the products with a healthy balance of fat, carbohydrate, protein, and calories per serving.

**Stouffer Family Size Dinners** offer restaurant caliber dishes baked in the **Family Cafe** oven.

*Family size boxes have calorie and nutrition information printed on the front of the box in large type.*

Chicken Alfredo = 280 calories per cup, 9g fat (3g saturated), 35g carbohydrate (fiber 2g, sugar 1g), 14g protein

Grandmas Chicken and Vegetable Rice Bake = 340 calories per ¼ package, 15g fat (5g saturated), 34g carbohydrate (fiber 1g, sugar 4g), 15g protein (easily increase to 6-8 servings lowering calories)

Lasagna with Meat & Sauce = 300 calories per cup, 10g fat (5g saturated), 16g carbohydrate (fiber 4g, sugar 7g), 18g protein *(High in protein and fiber but 5g saturated fat and 7g sugar)*

Escalloped Chicken & Noodles = 280 calories per cup, 12g fat (2g saturated), 28g carbohydrate (fiber 2g, sugar 2g), 15g protein

Lasagna Italiano = 250 calories per cup, 9g fat (4g saturated), 30g carbohydrate (fiber 3g, sugar 8g), 13g protein

Satisfying Servings Lasagna with Meat & Sauce = 230 calories per cup, 8g fat (4g saturated), 24g carbohydrate (fiber 2g, sugar 6g), 15g protein

Easily add side salad, canned vegetable, and fruit to complete the meal.

# Frozen Vegetables

**Bird's Eye** offers a multitude of frozen vegetable and vegetable meal options that are low in sodium.

Steamfresh Broccoli = 30 calories per cup 20mg sodium

Steamfresh Mixed Vegetables = 50 calories per cup 25mg sodium

Steamfresh Cut Green Beans = 30 calories per ⅔ cup 0mg sodium

Steamfresh Broccoli, Carrots, Cauliflower = 30 calories per cup 30mg sodium

Steamfresh Stir Fry Vegetables = 25 calories per cup 10mg sodium *(Add to Knorr Fiesta Sides Chicken Fried Rice)*

Steamfresh Light Seasoned Asian Medley = 60 calories per cup 290mg sodium

Voila! Garlic Chicken = 145 calories per cup 385mg sodium

Riced Cauliflower with Italian Cheese = 45 calories per ¾ cup 360mg sodium

Teriyaki Stir Fry Vegetables = 170 calories per cup cooked 540mg sodium *(Add to Knorr Fiesta Sides Teriyaki Rice)*

Steamfresh Brown and Wild Rice with Broccoli & Carrots= 150 calories per cup cooked 25mg sodium

**Create your own meal and recipe** by adding lean ground beef, canned chicken or tuna, a pasta selection, and Knorr Fiesta Sides to any Bird's Eye Vegetable or Medley. Use the Fat Secret App to calculate calories and nutritional information and add to saved meals.

Add Bird's Eye Vegetables to an omelette, Helper Meal, or Knorr Fiesta Sides.

Get creative combining different components to create your own special meals for the **Family Cafe**.

# Family Meals

### Chicken Casserole Preparation:

2 small cans cream of mushroom soup, 16 oz fat free sour cream, two 12 oz cans chunk chicken, little jar sliced mushrooms, 2 packages Reduced Fat Club Crackers, 1 stick light margarine

Melt butter and mix with 2 packages of crumbled club crackers. Use mix to coat the bottom and sides of 3 quart casserole dish (approximately 8.5x13.5 inches) leaving enough to cover the top of the finished dish.

Mix soup, sour cream, and drained chicken together thoroughly. Pour into casserole dish and spread out evenly. Top with sliced mushrooms (½ to 1 cup) and cover with leftover cracker crumbles.

Bake at 425 for 30 minutes or until bubbly hot.

2590 calories, 8 servings, 324 calories per serving

13.5g fat (2.5g saturated), 27g carbohydrates (fiber 1.5g, sugar 10g), 21g protein, 1152mg sodium

Add sweet peas, wheat roll, and baked potato to complete the meal.

### *Substitute 24 0z of Starkist Chunk Light Tuna in Water for Tuna Casserole.*

2409 calories, 8 servings, 301 calories per serving

11g fat (1.75g saturated), 27g carbohydrates (fiber 1.5g, sugar 10g), 19.5g protein, 942mg sodium

## Bowtie Spaghetti Preparation:

3 ¾ cups bowtie pasta, 1 lb lean ground beef, 2 green bell peppers, 2 red bell peppers, 1 large onion, 1-2 cups mushrooms, 1 large bottle Ragu Sauce, 1 can tomato paste, shredded fat free mozzarella cheese, 1 tomato

Start pasta boiling. Cut up vegetables. Brown ground beef and onion in healthy oil, season with garlic powder, salt, and pepper. Strain when done. Sauté vegetables in healthy oil and strain. Strain pasta, return to pot, add Ragu Sauce and tomato paste, stir and warm on medium heat. Add ground beef and vegetables, stir and continue to warm on medium heat for 10 minutes. Add sliced tomato and stir. Heat five more minutes. Top with shredded cheese.

3435 calories, 8 servings, 430 calories per serving

14.5g fat (4.5g saturated), 53g carbohydrates (fiber 10g, sugar 20g), 23.5g protein, 741mg sodium

## Linguine Spaghetti Preparation:

½ pack Ronco Spaghetti, 1 lb lean ground beef, 1 green bell pepper, 1 red bell pepper, 1 medium onion, 1-2 cups mushrooms, 1 large bottle Ragu Sauce, 1 can Hunts Tomato Sauce, 1 tomato

Season ground beef with tenderizer and let sit for ten minutes. Start pasta boiling. Cut up bell pepper into large chunks. Cut up onion. Brown ground beef in healthy oil, season with garlic powder, salt, and pepper, and add onion halfway thru cooking. Strain when done. Sauté bell pepper and mushrooms in healthy oil and strain. Strain pasta, return to pot, add Ragu Sauce and Hunt's Tomato Sauce, stir and warm on medium heat. Add ground beef and vegetables, stir and continue to warm on medium heat for 10 minutes. Add sliced tomato and stir. Heat five more minutes.

3395 calories, 8 servings, 425 calories per serving

14.5g fat (4.5g saturated), 53g carbohydrates (fiber 9.5g, sugar 18g), 20g protein, 1139mg sodium

**Substitute 12-16 medium meatballs for ground beef for Spaghetti and Meatballs.**

3162 calories, 8 servings, 395 calories per serving (16 meatballs)

11g fat (3g saturated), 57g carbohydrates (fiber 10g, sugar 19g), 17g protein, 1369mg sodium

## Pan Cooked Boneless Pork Chop & Sweet Potato Preparation:

2-4 sweet potatoes, 2-4 boneless lean pork chops, olive oil, vegetable oil, flour, Ziploc Bag, light margarine

Place 2-4 sweet potatoes in baking pan lined with aluminum foil and bake for 1 hour at 425. Consider splitting sweet potatoes, adding cinnamon sugar and light margarine after 30 minutes.

Place pork chops on plate and sprinkle both side with Adolph's Tenderizer and let sit for 30-45 minutes.

Preheat a nonstick pan with vegetable oil on medium - high heat. Put a small amount of flour in a large Ziploc Bag and seal. Pour enough olive oil over pork chops to coat. One at a time place pork chops in Ziploc Bag and coat with flour. How much depends on your personal taste. For a light coating shake off excess before removing from bag. Place pork chops in preheated pan on medium heat and let sit for 1-2 minutes before turning first time. Turn occasionally for about 8 minutes for 1 inch thick pork chops. Add 2 tablespoons of light margarine halfway thru cooking. Remove pork chops and place on plate covered with paper towel. Cover plate with aluminum foil and let sit 5 minutes. Add light margarine to sweet potatoes.

4 oz Pork Chop = 280 calories / 1 large sweet potato = 180 calories

Complete this meal with a Caesar Salad Kit (add a tomato and cucumber), Glory Great Northern Beans, and Texas Toast.

*Feel free to skip the flour step and cook in oil and light margarine.*

**Pan Seared Steak Preparation:**

Place steaks of choice on plate and sprinkle both side with Adolph's Tenderizer and let sit for 30-45 minutes. Preheat nonstick pan on high heat until water droplets roll around like little balls. Lightly coat pan with healthy oil. Place steaks in pan and let sit 1-2 minutes before turning. Wait 1-2 minutes before turning again. Turn heat to medium. Depending on the thickness of steak and desired doneness, cook 6-8 minutes (learn to use personal judgement in the moment of cooking). Adding 2 tablespoons of light margarine at halfway point is an option. Feel free to cut into the steak to check desired doneness. Remove steaks and place on plate covered with paper towel. Cover plate with aluminum foil and let sit 5 minutes.

**Pan cooked Hamburger Preparation:**

Place hamburgers on plate and sprinkle both side with Adolph's Tenderizer, brush both sides with Kraft Honey BBQ sauce and let sit for 30-45 minutes. For cheeseburgers place fat free cheese slices on counter to soften. Preheat nonstick pan lightly coated with healthy oil on high heat until oil starts to smoke and turn to medium. Place hamburgers in pan and season first side lightly with salt and pepper. Let sit 1-2 minutes before turning first time. Lightly season second side with salt and pepper. Cook 6-8 minutes turning occasionally until desired doneness. Feel free to cut into the hamburger to check the desired doneness. Add fat free cheese the final two minutes for cheeseburgers. Remove hamburgers and place on plate covered with paper towel. Cover plate with aluminum foil and let sit 5 minutes.

**Cooking meat in a pan should be a fluid endeavor** that seeks to get the best results with a particular piece of meat in the moment. Directions should always be seen as a guideline not rigid structure. As cooking skills progress raise or lower temperatures, adjust cooking times, and decide how often the meat should be turned.

Be creative and feel free to add seasoning, sauces, marinades, and vegetables to the cooking process.

**Salmon Patty Preparation:**

16 oz canned salmon, 2 eggs, ¼ cup fat free milk, ½ teaspoon salt, ⅛ teaspoon black pepper, ½ cup Reduced Fat Club Crackers

Preheat healthy oil on medium - high until hot then return to medium heat (for crisper patties cook on higher heat). Drain salmon and remove all skin and bones. Add beaten eggs, milk, and salmon together. Mix thoroughly and add seasoning and crumbled club crackers. Mix thoroughly and form into 6 patties. Patties will seem loose but, they will firm up immediately during cooking of first side. Drop by hand into skillet or use spatula to lift from plate into oil. Place patties in pan, turn after 1-2 minutes, and cook until golden brown on both sides.

901 calories, 6 servings, 150 calories per serving

6.5g fat (1.5g saturated), 2.5g carbohydrates (sugar 1g), 19g protein, 89mg sodium

Add cream potatoes, sweet peas, and a side salad to complete the meal.

*Top salmon patties with light maple syrup for a kick of flavor.*

## Family Size Lasagna Preparation:

16 oz lasagna pasta, 2 lbs lean ground beef, 8 oz fat free cream cheese, 12 oz tomato paste, shredded fat free mozzarella, garlic powder, onion, bell pepper, 3 quart (13.5x8.5) casserole dish

Prepare pasta and strain. Brown ground beef (seasoning with garlic powder), onion, and bell pepper. Mix meat, onion, bell pepper, cream cheese, and tomato paste. Do layer of pasta, layer of meat / sauce mixture, and top with shredded cheese. Then repeat. Bake in preheated oven at 400 for 15-20 minutes or until bubbly hot. Makes 8-12 servings. Reduce calories by using less pasta and ground beef.

4466 calories, 10 servings, 446 calories per serving

18.5g fat (7g saturated), 40g carbohydrates (sugar 5g), 26.5g protein, 288mg sodium

## Stove Top Pumpkin Pie Preparation:

5 eggs, 3 cups sugar, 6 heaping tablespoons of flour, 1 can of pumpkin, 4 cups fat free milk, 2 tablespoons of light margarine, nutmeg, cinnamon, 2 *Keebler Ready Crust Graham Pie Crust 2 Extra Serving* pie crusts (make sure to get the larger **2 Extra Serving** pie crusts). Makes 2 large pies.

Beat 1 egg, brush pie shells with egg, preheat oven to 375 and bake for 5 minutes. Set aside to cool.

Mix items thoroughly in order one at a time in a large bowl: Beat 4 eggs, gradually add 3 cups sugar and mix completely, add 6 heaping tablespoons of flour (more is better than less) and blend with mixer, add one can of pumpkin and mix, add 4 cups fat free milk and stir.

Empty bowl into stove top nonstick pot. Add 2 tablespoons light margarine and a light sprinkle of nutmeg and cinnamon. Start out with heat on medium. Stir continuously until sugar begins to clump and turn to low heat. Cook 16-20 minutes stirring the entire time. Do not leave unattended. Look for it to pop like lava and thicken without clumping to be ready to pour into pie shells. Pour evenly until both pie shells are full. Use a large spatula, spoon, or stirring tool to smooth and swirl the top of each pie from the outside to the center of the pie. Let cool on countertop for one hour. Replace pie crust covers and refrigerate for 24 hours.

3172 calories per pie, 10 servings, 317 calories per serving

7.5g fat (4g saturated), 57g carbohydrates (fiber 1g, sugar 40g), 3.5g protein, 49mg sodium

This is a guilty pleasure probably only indulged in at Thanksgiving and Christmas.

# Fresh from the Grill

Get a grill, buy some charcoal, and fire it up. Try to buy a grill with an adjustable shelf on each side and the front to provide workspace for cooking. Purchase more than one type of tongs for adjusting coal briquettes and food. Consider obtaining a grill pan to place on top of the grill grate so that smaller food items will not fall thru to the fire. This pan will prevent flair ups and make for easier cleanup. Cover the entire grill bowel and charcoal pan with aluminum foil. Simply throw away the aluminum foil instead of extensive cleaning. Spray the grill grate and grill pan with Pam before grilling. Get a brush for applying marinade and sauces. Look for a properly sized grill cover, if the grill will be left out in the elements. Find a multi utility lighter for starting the fire. Consider Matchlight charcoal instead of using lighter fluid. Buy a utility wire brush for cleaning the grill grate.

Start with a pile of 12-18 briquettes and light. Let coals burn until they are white hot. Spread coals evenly over bottom of the grill and adjust the height of the grill grate food will be placed on. If equipped with vents open halfway adjusting based on personal tastes and experience. Spray grill grate and grill pan with Pam.

Try Kraft Honey BBQ Sauce as your marinade. Brush onto hamburgers, hotdogs, vegetable skewers, and corn on the cob. One the selected items have been brushed close the lid and wait 5 minute before turning and brushing with BBQ sauce. Continue this process and remove items as they are done. Place on a plate lined with a paper towel. Cover the plate with aluminum foil until ready to eat.

Tenderize and marinate steaks before placing on the grill. Try different methods of preparation and marinades based on the type of steak being cooked, the occasion, and personal tastes. Continue marinating the steak while grilling.

Look for chicken or beef vegetable skewers at the local grocery store. Create colorful tasty skewers for the grill that include: red bell peppers, onions, green bell peppers, tomatoes, yellow bell peppers, mushrooms, and squash. Brush with Kraft Honey BBQ sauce. Look for jumbo shrimp in the frozen section that are already cooked and add between the vegetables. Brush shrimp with melted butter.

Build a boat from aluminum foil and place on the grill. Fill with shrimp and cover in melted butter.

The possibilities are endless. Pork chops, chicken, and ribs are just a few of the additional items to be tried on the grill. ***Make it an event with friends, children, pets, and music.***

# Snacks

Try to keep a wide range of low calorie satisfying snack items in the pantry. Here are is a small sample of the choices available. Each of these selections should be 200 calories or less.

**Fruit**: apple, orange, pear, banana, grapes, raisins

**Canned Fruit in Light Syrup:** peaches, pears, pineapple

**Dry Cereal:** Reese's Puffs, Captain Crunch, Cinnamon Toast Crunch (1 cup serving of cereal of choice)

**Breakfast Items**: 1 cereal bar, 1 pop tart

**Reduced Fat Crackers:** Cheez-Its, Wheat Thins, Club Crackers, Ritz Crackers (1 serving)

**Sweet:** 60 calorie Pudding Cup, 60 calorie Activia Yogurt, 40 calorie Hershey Mini Candy Bar, strawberries with whipped cream

# 8 Learn to Shop

*Follow these guidelines for grocery shipping:*

1. Create a specific meal plan for breakfast, lunch, dinner, and snacks.

2. Make a list of the items needed for the week's meals.

3. Include the foods that will be snacks throughout the day.

4. Buy only items that are on this list.

5. Shop when there is time to read labels and compare caloric, nutritional and the economic value of the products purchased.

6. Do not impulse shop.

7. Be prepared to shop at more than one store to obtain the low calorie and low fat items needed to fill out the week's meal plan.

8. Shop with the attitude of buying fresh, healthy, and happy foods.

## The Grocery List

Download an app that will create a grocery list template that allows you to check the items needed for a given week. Pen and paper work just as well. Divide the list based on areas or aisles of the store rather than a random order. Start with the part of the store where shopping will begin. Stores are laid out differently so base the list on the layout of the primary store that will be frequented.

The function of the list is to purchase products that are part of a weekly meal plan rather than being led by impulse. Once the serving size, calories per serving, and nutritional information of a given product fall within the meal plan and calorie goal, the process of shopping will speed up. Products and their availability change weekly. Any new product or food item with different serving size, calories per serving, or nutritional information will need to be examined label by label to see how it fits into the meal plan and daily calorie goal.

## Read Labels with Blind Eye

Feel free to peruse items not on the list and consider how they might liven up the weekly meal plan. Look at any item with a blind eye to what it is and look at **what combination of macros** it contains. It could be high in fat but, how much is saturated fat or even the bad trans fat? Maybe it is high in carbohydrates but, how many grams of fiber and sugar make up the total? Does it contain an adequate amount of protein and how many milligrams of sodium are in a single serving? What is the serving size, how many calories in a serving, and how does this compare to other food items already on the meal plan?

Try not to be tempted by a combination of the ads seen on TV combined with product packaging. Just because something doesn't have trans fat or is low in sugar doesn't necessarily make it healthy or right for the meal plan. Manufacturers only goal is to get the consumer to buy their product whether it is healthy, economical, or right for their lifestyle.

## Economics

Whether Walmart is your store of choice or not, the bottom line when shopping for a large load of groceries: It is hard or impossible to beat the cost savings obtained there. Walmart, also, tends to carry most of the low fat and low calories items on a given list. This being said, Walmart may not carry the particular low calorie or low fat item that will fill out the weeks's grocery list. Make the effort to discover which stores carry the particular items required to meet the daily calorie goal.

The larger size of many items may be cost effective when comparing volume / quantity to price but, often two smaller versions of a product can be the better buy. The 26 oz box of Product X might cost $4.50 (17.3 cents per oz), while two 15 oz boxes cost $4.75 (15.8 cents per oz).

Remember that convenience and drugstore grocery prices are always higher and often the items come in smaller quantities. Look for specials, sales, and coupons to getter cheaper prices at smaller stores and drugstores.

Dog food is a good example of buying in large quantity. The 28-32 lb bag of dog food is always going to be the economical way to go. The smaller the quantity, the higher the cost per pound, especially at a drugstore.

Rawhide chews are a wonderful way to keep your dog occupied, happy, and healthy. As a rule, I try, to spend less than 1 dollar per rawhide chew. Walmart has the best price and variety when looking for a rawhide chew. The price per chew at any other store is 2-3 times higher, especially pet stores.

To drive down the cost of the weekly grocery bill: Consider driving to a store in an area with lower sales tax, cutting coupons, for senior's groceries shop on senior discount day, and product comparison shopping (where the products have comparable nutritional and caloric value).

# Buy Fresh

In a grocery store the newest and freshest items are always on the bottom of a pile, stack, or the back of a shelf or freezer. Always take the time to find products with the latest usable date. A good rule of thumb on bread is 8-10 days. Milk should have a usable date of 10-14 days. Use common sense and how soon products are expected to be eaten when looking at dates on other products.

Take the time to look at each fruit or vegetable before buying: squeeze tomatoes for firmness, check the entire carton of strawberries, consider the color and look of the bananas, thump the watermelon, and handpick the bell peppers. Take the time to learn the signs of fresh, healthy fruits and vegetables.

When considering meat, look for lean cuts that are not filled with fat and have good marbling and texture. Once a variety of meats have been bought and cooked a feel for a quality piece of meat will become second nature.

If you do not see what you are looking for, ask for help or get the butcher to cut and package your specific request. The choices are varied and will come down to personal taste and what items will fit within the daily calorie goal.

# Healthy

Limit food items with caffeine. Excess caffeine can cause negative health effects like digestion issues, nervousness, irritability, inability to sleep, headache and other chronic symptoms. [8]

Whole grains and vegetables are an excellent source of complex carbohydrates. Add them to the weekly meal plan and daily calorie goal wherever possible. [4]

**Healthy Bread Shopping Tips:** 100% whole wheat flour listed as first ingredient, 2g fiber per slice, and less than 200 mg sodium per slice. [9]

Limit or eliminate products containing **trans fat**. Trans fat can be found in processed foods, crackers, cookies, margarine, and some salad dressings. [5]

Always look for a low fat, low sugar, low calorie option for any product on the weekly meal pan.

Try to resist items high in saturated fat and sugar. Especially high calorie, empty calorie items like desserts, sweets, pastries, and alcohol.

# Happy

Be creative and buy colorful interesting foods to prepare for the week's meals. Consider a new fruit, vegetable, lean meat, or pasta and vegetable dish to enliven mealtime. Eating should be as happy and fulfilling as any other part of your daily life. Take the time to stock the pantry with foods that are fun to prepare and an adventure to eat. Try shopping at a local farmer's market for home grown produce. Find a store that is a pleasure to visit and turn grocery shopping into an occasion.

# 9 Zen

Exercise - Activity - Involvement - Natural World

Getting moving is one of the most important aspects of a healthy lifestyle. Find ways to be active in your work, play, and recreation.

Any physical activity burns calories, increases metabolism, and will help reach and maintain a goal weight.

**Download the Exercise Calculator App**, enter weight, duration, and activity, to get calories burned.

Physical activity and exercise can be broken down into four categories: **Recreation, Fitness, Work, and Zen**.

A recreational activity is something done for fun and may require a certain setting, time frame, equipment, and participants. Here is a list of **recreational activities** that anyone can take an interest in learning.

*The calories burned by a 150 pound person after 30 minutes will be listed in parenthesis for each activity.*

Tennis (250), Racquetball (250), Ping Pong (143), Horseshoes (105)

Walk (107), Run (286), Hike (214), Climb (250), Bike (214), Fishing (107)

Football (321), Baseball (180), Softball (180), Basketball (286), Volleyball (143)

Canoe (143), Kayak (179), Sail (107), Water Ski (214), Surf (107)

Scuba Dive (250), Snorkel (179)

Skiing (250), Snowboarding (220)

Roller Blade (50), Roller Skate (425)

Bowling (107), Frisbee (107), Billiards (89), Darts(89)

Gardening (143), Fly a Kite (250)

Enjoying the day and the outdoors is as simple as picking up a frisbee, football, kite, or baseball.

Choose one new hobby and give it a try. Add something new to the weekly routine that expands the mind and gets the body moving.

Gather friends for group sports and activities, so that exercise becomes fellowship.

**These activities can be both recreational and fitness:**

Yoga (89), Pilate's (125)

Weight Training (107), Spin Class (250), Water Aerobics (200)

Bench Aerobics (230), Kick Boxing (250), Cardio Funk (200)

The best way to stay fit is to love doing an activity so much it is not thought of as exercise.

**Fitness:**

Walk (107), Run (286), Treadmill (110)

Spin Class (250), Any Aerobic Workout Machine (varies)

Bench Aerobics (230), Kick Boxing (250), Cardio Funk (200)

Yoga (89), Pilate's (125), Swim Laps (250), Water Aerobics (200)

Weight Training (107), Fitness Trainer (varies)

Working out, toning up, getting fit, are all ways of expressing a desire to look and feel our best. There is no reason it cannot be fun, interesting, and challenging. Find the right gym, trainer, class, course, or niche to sculpt the mind and body. There is a right place and a right fitness activity for everyone.

**Work:**

Housework (100), Yard work (161), Grocery Shopping (130)

Carpenter (107), Construction Worker (150), Landscaper (250)

Retail Sales (50), Restaurant Worker (85), Warehouse Stocking (varies)

Mechanic (60), Repairman (60), Teacher (varies)

This is just a sample of the jobs that are physically active. Go to **calorielab.com** or **Google** to find the results for a specific job.

The benefits of working a physically active job can be undone by poor eating and drinking habits. A physically demanding job, that burns calories, does not give anyone a license to eat an excess of high calorie, empty calorie, high fat, unhealthy food and drink. Eat enough healthy calories to adequately power the body thru the tasks of the day.

**Be creative** in finding ways to be active and burn extra calories. Chewing gum can burn 55 calories an hour and alleviate sinus and allergy symptoms (my personal experience). Go out and dance, walk up a flight of stairs, or play tug of war with your dogs. Anything that gets you moving and exerts an effort is burning calories and raising the heart rate.

***Play a video game!*** Yes, if you actually go thru the physical motions of the sport or activity being played on the Wii, the physical exertion will burn calories. Get out of the chair, off the couch, and swing the pseudo tennis racquet, baseball bat, bowling ball, golf club, and be active even if other activities are not an option.

**Get a good night's rest.** 7-9 hours of sleep allows for feeling good and making smart decisions. Deciding to follow the meal plan, getting some exercise, and choosing a good path come from a well rested brain and body.

# Your Zen

The Mahayana Buddhist view of Zen is a state of mind that focuses on one's intuition and meditation.

The Urban Dictionary defines Zen as state of focus where the mind and body are one; the things of the world are seen for what they are and not what our mind wants them to be.

Zen applies to physical activity and getting the body moving. It could be more than one category of physical activity but, it will be something done 5-6 days a week, hopefully outdoors. Your Zen is your own. It is not work, for fitness, or simply recreational; it gives balance in form of physical activity and communing with the natural world. Part of Zen will be connecting with the natural world if you have not already.

Zen also applies to where you live, work, relationships, fun, learning, growing, and expanding your personal boundaries. Every component in daily life is interconnected and should compliment each other. Focus on the whole of your daily life and not the individual pieces. See the whole of a puzzle to be able to assemble it.

My own experience has encompassed all four areas of physical activity. Many of the jobs I worked have been physically demanding with little or no time to sit. For years I belonged to a gym using the treadmill, taking bench, kick boxing, and cardio funk classes, swimming laps, and having a personal trainer to put me thru a weight workout. Recreation has taken me to the bottom of the ocean and the top of the trail. Tennis, ping pong, bowling, swimming, biking, racquetball, camping, billiards, scuba diving, and hiking are some of the activities that kept me busy at various times in my life.

My Zen now is walking my dogs, Kink and Bell. Yes, it's necessary because I live in an apartment, it's needed because it burns calories, and it is normally enjoyable but, it goes beyond that. The hikes and walks we take occur at every time of day, in every season, during every kind of weather, and we always discover something new. It is a way to connect with the natural world and commune. It is something I want to do and need to do to have balance. My Zen has helped free me from the roller coaster of losing and gaining weight.

Work, recreational activities, and fitness plans will come and go but, finding Your Zen can reshape the daily life. It's ok if the Zen changes as long as it stays part of the balance of a healthy lifestyle.

Walking is one of the best ways to be active, and the easiest. Taking a walk can be done anywhere, anytime, in any weather, or season, for any distance. What makes any walk better? Well, company of course! Especially, the companionship of dogs.

## Consider Adopting A Dog

Before ever contemplating adopting a dog, first determine if you have the characteristics and traits necessary to be a responsible, considerate, pack leading dog owner.

Here are some of the necessary requirements:

1. I am a responsible person that does not shirk my duties.

2. I am a respectful person to others in all situations

3. I am a respectful neighbor that considers how my actions affect the quality of life of those that live around my home / apartment.

4. I will make time to take my dog on a minimum of 3 to 4 walks, of at least 15 minutes, each every day.

5. I will take it upon myself to choose a breed, or mix breed of dog, that's characteristics fit with my current lifestyle.

6. I will consider my current work, living, and economic situation, before adopting a dog.

7. I will research methods of training and being pack leader before adopting a dog.

8. I will plan on training my dog to be well behaved on a leash.

9. I will plan on walking my dog on a leash at all times.

10. I will not leave my dog out in a yard, or on a patio all day, to bark and bother my neighbors.

11. I will not cage or chain up my dog in lieu of training and proper care.

12. I will learn to walk my dog properly on a leash, be respectful of others walking their dog, and try to give way or walk a different direction, to allow others the same right to take their dog for a walk.

13. I will make sure my dog gets all shots and medical treatment needed to be a healthy, happy dog.

14. I will feed my dog healthy dog food, and limit treats and other sources of food, to ensure my dogs stay at a healthy weight.

15. I will spend the first year actively being the pack leader, training my dog, and setting my dog up for success when left alone in a house or apartment.

16. I will work to see my dog leads an interesting fulfilling life.

17. When it is time, I will have my dog spade or neutered.

18. I understand that my dog will need love and companionship, and will not abandon the dog to a yard or basement because the cute puppy phase is over.

19. I understand puppies grow up to be dogs that require full time care.

20. I will take full responsibility for my dog's actions and take the blame for any missteps due to lack of training or pack leadership.

21. I will try to adopt a dog first before supporting the breeding industry.

22. I will secure my home / apartment and yard before adopting a puppy or dog.

Kink and Bell are my Zen. They have brought peace, harmony, and unconditional love into my life. Walking my dogs healed a chronic sciatic nerve pain issue I had suffered with for 2 years. The daily exercise has allowed me to get off the weight gain and loss carousel.

The right dog, that is planned and prepared for, can change the fabric and Zen of anyone's life; if the 22 points stated above are used as a framework, for what it means to be a dog owner.

If you do have a house, make sure there is a place to walk your dog, whether it's the neighborhood, a park, or a trail. Being lazy and letting the dog out in the yard, in lieu of walking, deprives the dog and you of exercise and adventure.

Find a place to take a 45 minute to an hour hike 3-5 times a week. Pile in the car and make an excursion out of it. Get away from roads, cars, people, and distractions of an urban jungle. Go back to the natural world.

# Natural World

Make time to enjoy the natural world everyday. The best part is that it is free!

Ten days out of every month, the moon is visible during the daytime. Look for the daytime moon and hawks soaring on rising currents. Watch the cloud formations in the sky and the world reflected in the waters. Take five minutes each day to feel the sun on your face and give thanks for feeling the warmth of the world and life.

Always watch the sunset each and everyday. Look for the phases of the moon, constellations like Orion and the Big Dipper, and visible planets like Mars or Venus. Download the **Google Sky App** to learn and find specific objects in the night sky.

Notice the plants, flowers, and trees around you. The buzzing of a bee, the sweet song of a bird, the rustle of a squirrel, or the hovering of a hummingbird.

The natural world is the real world. It is where peace, harmony, and balance can come from daily.

If need be, get in the car, and drive or walk where the peace and quiet of nature can be observed.

***In the spirit of the natural world, Do Not Liter.*** Leave behind footprints not bottle caps, wrappers, cigarette butts, water bottles, and the myriad of trash the urban world creates and caries with it everywhere. The trash you are too lazy to throw away will spoil someone else's walk.

Revel in anytime that can be spent in the natural world. Share it, photograph it, write about it, and respect it.

# 10 Understand the Relationship

Between Exercise, Counting Calories, and a Goal Weight

Counting calories, exercise, or a combination can be used to to reach a goal weight.

Simply counting calories based on the ADCC and a Daily Calorie Goal will result in weight loss or maintenance.

Relying on a strenuous fitness routine to burn the calories needed to maintain a goal weight is also possible.

These two methods of weight loss and maintenance can work but, are usually doomed to fail by themselves. True freedom is the marrying of these two disciplines into a symbiotic relationship.

## Exercise

Dedication, routine, and finding your Zen can lead to a pattern of physical activity that is beneficial and healthy. The realities of life, work, family, illness, inclement weather, and overriding responsibilities will ultimately lead to periods of inactivity. These periods of inactivity will see a drop in metabolism and daily calories burned. This drop in calories burned with no concern for calories consumed can lead to weight gain and backsliding.

## Counting Calories

Despite knowing your kryptonite, yearly cycle, high calorie obstacles, and what to look for on each and every label; there will be a time when "eat, drink, and be merry" is the theme of the day, week, and month.

During this period without a way to burn off extra calories, weight may be gained and a general backslide occurs.

# Symbiosis

Counting calories and eating healthy, insures that during times of inactivity more frugality may be used in weekly and daily meal plans to insure weight gain does not occur.

A daily routine that incorporates physical activity allows for an increase in the time spent and calories burned. This increase can offset a period of "eat, drink, and be merry."

# Benefits

The benefits of this symbiosis can be seen in lowering risk factors for disease, stress, depression, weight gain, and insomnia; increasing contentment, happiness, well being, energy, motivation, positivity, self image, rest, relaxation, and a State of Zen.

Learn to eat the same foods for less calories. Find your Zen and get moving in the natural world. Find a balance in everyday living.

# 11 Create a Space

Be a Part of the Natural World
*Eat, Play, Rest, Meditate*

Create a space in the natural world to grill, eat, play, rest, meditate, and enjoy the beauty of the day. Almost everyone has a natural space that can be used to bring everyday life outside. Whether it is large or small, private or open, covered or open to the elements, utilize any porch, patio, or grassy space for living everyday life.

## Covered Outdoor Spaces

Get some rugs. There is nothing like a rug to give a space the feel of a room. Regardless of the size of the patio or porch, inexpensive, colorful rugs, that will fit your décor can be found at a myriad of discount stores.

Find the right padded folding chairs and make a place to sit. Add one or more outdoor tables and coasters to create space for eating, drinking, working, and relaxing.

Incorporate the grill of your choice into the layout. Run an extension cord under a door or thru a window, and a add a power strip to provide electricity for all needs.

Hang wind chimes, Hummingbird feeders, signs, and memorabilia suitable for an outdoor space. Laminate any paper items, photos, pictures, or artwork to protect from the elements and make suitable for hanging in an outside environment. From small to large, anything can be laminated in a clear plastic sleeve at FedX Kinko's. Use wood frames without glass or laminate items already mounted on matt board. Use industrial double-sided tape where nails / screws will not work.

Consider hanging a thin tapestry on a wall using the industrial double-sided tape. Use street signs, personalized license plates, Coca Cola signs, or anything that fits your personal tastes and style.

Use candles, glass containers, rocks, crystals, and baskets to create different focal points, niches, and areas of peace and beauty throughout the space.

Reuse items instead of putting in the trash. Rust-Oleum spray paint can turn almost anything old and outdated into something fresh and new. Paint a table, chair, plant stand, watering can, grill, or any object so that it can find a new unique purpose, other than the trash heap.

One great example is the large, solid, round piece of glass found in a microwave. When I had to purchase a new microwave, the glass from the old microwave made the perfect top to an old plastic table. The old, scarred white table got a new coat of gloss black paint. The glass fit perfectly, creating a glass tabletop, and something new from two items that could have been sent to the landfill.

Shopping at the local Dollar Store is an inexpensive way to decorate any porch or patio. Fake fruit, frames, candles, glass vases and containers of all shapes and sizes, pottery, plates, glasses, wind chimes, pots, spades, and any number of things can be found for $1. There is often replica artwork ($1) that can be laminated ($1) and framed ($1) for as little as $3.

Pot some plants, flowers, and ferns to bring life and color to the outdoor space.

Repot **ferns** into hanging baskets with muslin and extra potting soil to allow for growth.

**Geraniums** are one of the best blooming plants and will last the entire season. Take the time to pinch off old blooms, so the plant will continue to flower and not go into a dormant phase.

**Begonias** are another blooming plant, that come in a variety of colors, and will bloom the entire season. They make great hanging pots.

**Caladium** colors can be mixed into as large or small a pot that is desired.

**Vinca** need sunlight, come in many colors, and bloom prolifically.

**New Guinea Impatiens** are colorful with large blooms, need several hours of sun a day but, may need to be watered everyday to insure they do not wilt.

Also, consider potting plants that will be kept year round by moving them inside for the winter months.

Use different size, color, texture, and types of pots for visual interest. Incorporate plant stands for individual and multiple plant use. Create your very own jungle or secret garden.

Two of my favorite types of plant to combine and use on a patio are Mother-In-Law Tongues and almost any type of cactus. Creating mixed pots will bring interest to the space by providing an ever changing landscape.

Consider potting and creating your own pineapple plant. Simply go to the grocery store and look for the greenest pineapple with large green foliage coming out of the top of the fruit. Cut the top off the pineapple about two inches below the foliage. Pot the meaty part of the cutting below the soil, leaving the foliage sticking up. Wait several days and water sparingly. It will take awhile to root. If the first attempt is unsuccessful try again. Once rooted the plant needs ample sunlight and within a year will be significantly larger. Repot as the plant outgrows it's space. This will provide a big, beautiful plant not found many places except Hawaii. Every 2.5 years it will bear a fruit that can be transplanted to create an offspring plant.

The first rule with plants is to always use pots that drain and do not over water. Less is always more when it comes to watering plants. If unsure, go by the directions that came with the plant when it was purchased, or simply Google it.

Miracle-Gro can be added to watering ever 10-14 days when temperatures are not over 85 degrees. Miracle-Gro will stimulate growth, so be prepared to water plants as needed within a day or two of use. Use Miracle-Gro potting soil to see amazing results from all potted plants.

Be careful where plants are placed, and how much direct sunlight they will receive. Unless specifically stated, most plants do not need direct sunlight. A plant that does not do well in direct sun can burn up quickly if placed in the sun. Do not be afraid to make mistakes. Growing and caring for plants is a continual learning process. Plants, like dogs, will bring peace and joy to your daily life.

## Open or Grassy Spaces

For the **open patio,** consider a large umbrella for shade, and a grill cover to protect from the elements. Add chairs and tables to facilitate outdoor living. Unless weather safe, remember to fold up and stow away patio items during storms.

**Grassy spaces** should always be reveled in each and every day. Buy an inexpensive bench, simple side table, and sit in your own private park.

Pitch a tent and create the family campground. Add a fire pit and enjoy the outdoors at night. Get a horseshoe set and set up a pit. Use rocks and wood chips to create beds around trees and plant groupings. Hang bird-houses and Hummingbird feeders. Throw a frisbee, football, baseball, or dog's ball. Get a Bluetooth speaker and enjoy the tunes of your choice.

Find balance in natural world: meditate, exercise, eat, think, read, listen, observe, revel, enjoy, work, contemplate, and relax.

## 12 Find a Balance

Mind, Body, and Spirit

Ultimately, to be successful in living a healthy happy life, there must be balance. What is the source and inspiration for this balance?

## Ordered Universe

Since the first man and woman looked at the natural world in awe of the infinite diversity in infinite combinations, cast their eyes to the stars in wonderment at what the heavens hold, and marveled at the creation of life everyday; man has looked for an order to the universe.

The world we know, and the universe that is explored, is organized from the galaxies containing millions of stars, down to the protons, neutrons, and electrons at the subatomic level. The cells that form all living things organize themselves and change spontaneously to create the systems, bones, skin, eyes, wings, leaves, branches, scales, feathers, feelers, claws, blooms, flowers, and intelligence necessary for each life form to live, reproduce, and thrive.

Across the planet are a myriad of interconnected ecosystems balanced for all living things. The energy for these systems comes from the sun. This sunlight is converted by plants, through photosynthesis, as well as capturing carbon dioxide and releasing oxygen. Plants are eaten by animals, the animals eat animals, and the dead plants and animals decompose, releasing carbon dioxide into the atmosphere to continue the nutrient cycle. This is a combination of the organic and non organic working in symbiosis.

On a planetary scale, there is a system of ocean currents driven by the Earth's rotation, wind, tides, and the sun. This circulation system transfers energy around the world, affecting weather, temperature, the recycling of

128

gas, and the movement of nutrients necessary for feeding the larva of marine ecosystems. These currents provide for stable weather and climate patterns. This conveyor belt moves warm, less dense water away from the equator and carries colder, denser water away from the poles toward the equator. [11]

The moon is exactly 400 times smaller than the sun. The sun is exactly 400 times farther from the earth than the moon. This allows for a perfect eclipse. How the moon was formed and ended up in just the right orbit around our planet is still up for debate and conjecture. The Apollo 12 Mission deliberately crashed the ascent stage of the Lunar Module into the surface of the moon. The seismometers that were installed between 1972-1977 recorded the moon ringing like a bell as if it were hollow. This beautiful, captivating object, also affects the tides.

In our solar system round planets revolve in orbit around the sun. Some of these planets are in turn circled by one or more moons of their own. Our solar system revolves around the center of the Milky Way Galaxy.

From the DNA in living organism, water flowing down a drain, the arms of the Milky Way Galaxy, the shells of animals, a sunflower head, the human fingerprint, and the cross section of a cabbage, the spiral shape is found throughout the natural world and the universe. The spiral is a specific geometric shape that can be expressed mathematically. This curve runs around a central point in an organized fashion.

The human body is run by chemical processes. Food is digested, energy is produced, and new cells are created thru division containing a copy of the genetic code. This is accomplished using the 75,000 enzymes in the human body. The process of this chemical reaction is best described as a lock and key. Each enzyme will only fit a certain lock starting a specific chemical reaction. The complexity of the chemical processes required to run the systems of a human body capable of thought, interaction, self awareness, creativity, reproduction, movement, and love, staggers the mind. [12]

There are 950,000 species of insects, 310,000  known animal species (10,000 added per year), and 325,00 plant species; all with their own genetic code and complex life processes. 13

Observations by PLANET (Probing Lensing Anomalies Network) have given a rough estimate of the possibility of 10 billion terrestrial planets across the Milky Way. Astronomers estimate **2 trillion** galaxies in the universe. These planets all revolve around stars that form solar systems. These solar systems revolve around galaxies. The galaxies fill the universe.

Everywhere man can explore from the subatomic level, the plants and animals in our ecosystems, to the planets, stars, and galaxies that make up the universe, there is a logical, scientific, common sense ordering of everything.

How could all of these complex systems, from atoms, the human body, Planet Earth, and the Milky Way Galaxy, have come from an explosion of matter and evolved into the ordered, colorful, creative, thought provoking, logical, renewing universe we live in today?

Across our world and thru time, man has considered this universe to have been created and ordered by a Supreme Being. The names for this organizing creative force have taken many names and spawned numerous religions.

Is it more logical to explain an ordered complex universe by intelligent design, or does a random evolution of everything, from the atom, human DNA, astronomical bodies, water currents, ecosystems, and the symbiosis of the organic and non organic, really make any sense?

## Who is the Intelligent Designer?

I believe the universe and everything in it was created and organized by a Supreme Being. This Supreme Being can be called God. He took great care in creating a universe with infinite diversity in infinite combinations. How long did this take? Genesis says seven days but, what is a day to God; 1000 years, 1 million years, 100 million years? We don't know how long it took to create the universe but, we are just starting to grasp the complexity and inter connectivity of everything everywhere.

What do we call this Supreme Being? What is His name? How will I know Him? When will I hear His voice?

# I AM that I AM

## The Exodus Story

Here is the story of Moses taken from the Book of Exodus in the NIV translation of the Bible.

Moses was an Israelite that lived from 1400 BCE to 1200 BCE in and around Egypt. He was born at a time when the enslaved Israelites had multiplied and become so numerous that the Egyptian Pharaoh decided all newborn male babies should be put to death. Mose's mother, Jochebed, hid him and spared his life. When the baby could no longer be hidden, she instructed her daughter Miriam to place him in a papyrus basket sealed with tar and pitch and let him float on the Nile. Miriam followed the basket through the reeds until it was discovered by the pharaoh's daughter. Miriam came up out of the river and asked if she should get a Hebrew woman to nurse the child. Jochebed nursed him and after a time he was taken to live as the pharaoh's daughter's son. He was called Moses since she drew him from the water.

Moses saw the affliction of his people in bondage and even killed an Egyptian that was beating a Hebrew slave. He hid the body but, the knowledge of what he had done became known. The pharaoh tried to have Moses killed so, he fled across the desert to Midian. It was there he tended sheep next to Mt. Horeb. The shepherds called Horeb, God's mountain.

One day Moses saw a bush on the mountain that was on fire, but did not burn. He wanted to go see this mysterious sight. It was then, for the first

131

time, Moses heard a soft voice call out to him. Moses replied, "Here I am." The voice told Moses to take off his sandals because he was on Holy Ground; He had seen the affliction of his people in Egyptian bondage and was sending Moses to bring them out of Egypt.

Moses asked why he should be sent and who should he say sent him. The voice replied, "I will be with you; I am the God of your father, the God of Abraham, the God of Isaac, and the God of Jacob."

Moses inquired of the voice,"What if I tell them the God of your fathers's has sent me and they ask what is His name?"

The voice replied, "I AM that I AM, tell them I AM has sent you."

It took me till later in life to grasp the concept of a God so large, so encompassing, so eternal, the Alpha, the Omega, the God of every star, blade of grass, living creature, creative thought, all light, and life, that He could not have a name. There is no way to name or define the power and depth of God other than to say, "I AM has sent me."

This assures us that all is in I AM's hands, at every moment, for all time. We may not know God just as Moses did not. We may not want to be called, as Moses did not. We may think we do not have the skills and abilities to do what we are called to do, just as Moses doubted his own worth but, God will give each man or woman the things needed to accomplish great things in this life.

## Automatons

A Supreme Being could have created organized, ordered, living beings, that did not disrupt the natural order. These beings would not truly have been sentient or filled the Supreme Being's void.

God gave man the gift of freewill. The right to choose. Even the ability to choose not to believe in a Supreme Being, God, or I AM. This is the same freewill you can use to lead a happy, healthy, productive life. A happy, healthy lifestyle is but one side of the coin. We are free to choose any path but, there will always be consequences.

God knew this and gave us freewill anyway. If we choose to believe in I AM we can call on him to help us with our decisions. The Bible can be used as a guidebook for navigating the universe and the complexity of freewill.

Do I have to join a church? Do I have to talk to a preacher? How do I learn about the Supreme Being I believe created an ordered logical universe?

Just like the plan you created using this book to reach and maintain a goal weight, Find Your Zen, and strive for balance; you can forge a personal relationship with the Supreme Being, God, or I AM. This relationship only requires three things: faith I AM created the universe, willingness to talk via prayer to God, and taking time to read the Bible using the Bible App and whichever translation appeals to your personal tastes.

Start by reading what appeals and sparks an interest. The Bible App contains explanations of scriptures and passages by everyday people. Prayer is simply talking in your head or out loud. Faith is something you have or don't have today.

Once a personal relationship with I AM is forged, and His inspired word has been contemplated, a foundation for balance can be established.

# Eternal Life

If there is a belief in a Supreme Being, if a relationship and study of I Am's word has been started, then the next logical question would be what happens when people die, loved ones die, or I die?

I AM gave us freewill. Unfortunately, all of us, save one, have chosen to sin. This sin takes many forms and God cannot look at or accept it. The wages of this sin should be death and punishment.

From the beginning, before the universe took form, when there was nothing but a formless void, I AM's son was with Him. God loved His son but, God loved us more. He chose to send His Son, in human form, to Earth to live as a man. This man would have the same frail body and the same freewill. This man was called Jesus and he lived in Galilee, worked as a carpenter, ate, drank, and slept as a man for 30 years.

Jesus was without sin and chose to do the will of God. He chose to minister to the sick, blind, poor, downtrodden, and outcast. This three year ministry can be found detailed in the New Testament of the Bible.

Many believed in Him and the words He spoke. Others feared and reviled Him. When the time came, His own people said, "Crucify Him." He was beaten, humiliated, and crucified on a wooden cross. Jesus had the power to save Himself. He could have cursed those that had crucified Him.

Instead Jesus, the sinless, bore the suffering and pain that should have been ours to bear. He forgave those that would not believe in Him and killed Him. He died, was buried, laid in a tomb sealed with a great stone, and guarded by those who feared His body would be stolen. Jesus had preached to believe in Him was to have everlasting life and to be forgiven of sins. It was said He would rise from the dead. The heavy stone and the soldiers were there to prevent the body from being stolen and a myth perpetuated.

On the third day after Jesus death, Mary went to the tomb and found the stone rolled away and the tomb empty. A man dressed in all white told her not to be alarmed. "The man you are looking for, Jesus of Nazarene, Is Risen!", he said.

The carpenter from Galilee, the minister to the sick and downtrodden, the sinless man reviled and crucified, the Son of I AM that always had been and always would be; fulfilled the prophecies of the Old Testament, and His own promise to return, to Arise on the third day, so that whosoever should believe on Him should nor perish, but have everlasting life.

You don't have to go to a church, talk to a pastor, do good works, or choose a specific religion or denomination to know Jesus. All you have to do is believe in a Supreme Being that created an ordered, logical universe, gave us freewill, and chose to give up His son Jesus; so that sinful freewill would not lead to our death and punishment.

If you believe in Jesus and are willing to repent of the daily sins committed, then you are saved. This new awareness brings the responsibility of living a different life. We are saved by Grace. We have all sinned but, we can choose to try and not sin, to live a happy, healthy life, and to help others do the same.

# Balance

Creating a plan to *Live Your Life, Forget the Diet, Find Your Zen* enables you to reach a goal weight, maintain that weight, be physically active each day, and live a healthy, happy daily life. This brings the body into balance.

The simple fact, that you created and executed a plan, that allows for living and enjoying life thru moderation and planning means the choices made are yours. The freedom to choose, being happy with the choices, and a balanced healthy body brings the mind into balance.

The knowledge that the universe, world, and ourselves were organized and created by a Supreme Being that loves us, cares for us, and provided for our eternal life, gives the spirit balance.

God does not promise us a life without trial, tribulation, and strife. He does promise to provide, protect, counsel, heal, restore, renew, and deliver us, if we humble ourselves to Him.

It takes work to have a balanced mind, body, and spirit. The natural world that I AM created is there to give peace, quiet, and wonderment.

Now that there is balance in ourselves, we can balance the ecosystem that is life. Don't look at the components in life like the juggler's balls; waiting to see which ball drops to the ground first. Each component should balance the others.

If possible find a job or work that can be enjoyed, looked forward to, and even reveled in each day. Find something fulfilling to pay the bills, not just a way to survive the month. Work, even if it is a calling, a Zen, should not be all encompassing, or an obsession. Work should not take away from recreation, play, rest, or Your Zen exercise. It should not keep you from family, friends, and responsibilities. Make choices with work daily and set up boundaries the same way smart choices are made about living a healthy lifestyle.

Find a place to live that is your own. A home should be a place of respite, quiet, security, peace, beauty, rest, and recreation. If home is not a happy place, then finding motivation and balance will be difficult. Decide what makes living worthwhile to you and seek out a place to live that fulfills those dreams. Create an outdoor space and enjoy the natural world.

Find love and embrace family, friends, and pets. Make time for the people that are important each and every day. Remember to hug, pet, kiss, talk to, embrace, play with, and share the day with others. Relationships are the true motivation in life.

Life is work. Life is play. Life is infinite diversity in infinite combinations. Find **Your Zen** in play, work, home, and relationships.

Find equal parts of loving, laughing, working, striving, dreaming, and loving. This is balance.

# Scriptures of Balance

**Romans 8:28 NIV**

And we know that in all things God works for the good of those who love him, who have been called according to his purpose.

**Psalm 23 NIV**

A psalm of David.

The Lord is my shepherd, I lack nothing. He makes me lie down in green pastures, he leads me beside quiet waters, he refreshes my soul.

He guides me along the right paths for his name's sake. Even though I walk through the darkest valley, I will fear no evil, for you are with me; your rod and your staff, they comfort me.

You prepare a table before me in the presence of my enemies. You anoint my head with oil; my cup overflows.

Surely your goodness and love will follow me all the days of my life, and I will dwell in the house of the Lord forever.

**Matthew 6:25-34 NIV**

Do Not Worry

Therefore I tell you, do not worry about your life, what you will eat or drink; or about your body, what you will wear.

Is not life more than food, and the body more than clothes? Look at the birds of the air; they do not sow or reap or store away in barns, and yet your heavenly Father feeds them. Are you not much more valuable than they? Can any one of you by worrying add a single hour to your life?

And why do you worry about clothes? See how the flowers of the field grow. They do not labor or spin. Yet I tell you that not even Solomon in all his splendor was dressed like one of these. If that is how God clothes the grass of the field, which is here today and tomorrow is thrown into the fire, will he not much more clothe you—you of little faith?

So do not worry, saying, "What shall we eat?" or "What shall we drink?" or "What shall we wear?". For the pagans run after all these things, and your heavenly Father knows that you need them. But seek first his kingdom and his righteousness, and all these things will be given to you as well.

***Therefore, do not worry about tomorrow, for tomorrow will worry about itself. Each day has enough trouble of its own.***

### John 3:16 NIV

For God so loved the world that he gave his one and only Son, that whoever believes in him shall not perish but have eternal life.

### 1 Corinthians 13:4-8 NIV

Love is patient, love is kind. It does not envy, it does not boast, it is not proud.

It does not dishonor others, it is not self-seeking, it is not easily angered, it keeps no record of wrongs.

Love does not delight in evil but rejoices with the truth. It always protects, always trusts, always hopes, always perseveres.

Love never fails.

# 13 How do I maintain?

Normally, when anyone loses weight, there is a period of bliss and excitement: the thrill of looking in the mirror, wearing new clothes, enjoying the compliments of accomplishment, and taking a break from the strenuous diet and exercise that has been a daily regimen.

This relief and abandonment of a regimen comes from an imbalance of mind, body, and spirit that leads right back to the roller coaster of weight gain and weight loss most people find themselves riding.

The plan, created and implemented from the tools and information in this book, lead to a change of lifestyle and mental awareness. The symbiosis of counting calories / eating healthy and daily physical activity is the key to maintenance

The ability to eat the same foods, but consume less calories, planning for the Daily Quotient and Eating Events, Finding Your Zen when it comes to exercise, and looking at all food and drink differently, is not strenuous or a difficult. These choices lead to an everyday life that is enjoyed, anticipated, and balanced.

The plan, your plan, has maintenance already built in, because you are able to *Live Your Life, Forget the Diet, Find Your Zen.*

# 14 What if I backslide?

It's OK! Life is an ebb and flow. It is easy to resume buying low calorie foods, cutting calories, and getting daily exercise without a big resolution.

*The best part is this is your plan.* Reexamine the **Daily Quotient** and where it fell short. Be truthful about what your **Kryptonite** is and whether it has been avoided. Consider the meal plan and the foods chosen. Are there low calorie, low fat, sugar free options for items in the weekly meal plan? Did you identify and account for **Your Yearly Cycle**? Have you found **Your Zen**? Is the symbiosis of counting calories / eating healthy and daily physical activity being utilized?

The key to success is being truthful with yourself. Identify the obstacles that have hindered reaching a weight loss goal or maintaining a goal weight. Utilize the information and tools in this book to start a new plan that is honest and ready for change.

*Remember it is simple math:*

Eat 500 calories less per day to lose one pound per week.

Based on the **ADCC** and the level of **Physical Activity** eat the same amount of calories that are burned each day to maintain the current weight.

*Find balance in life:* equal parts of playing, working, eating, family, friends, growth, experience, and happiness.

Look for **Your Zen** and commune with the natural world. Find Zen in all parts of your life.

**Everyone** can reach and maintain a goal weight that makes them feel happy in their own skin. **Good Luck!**

# Glossary of Terms

**ADCC** or **A**verage **D**aily **C**alorie **C**onsumption is the total calories for a time frame divided by the days in the time frame.

The number from the first weigh in is a **baseline**.

Weighing on your **baseline scale** gives the most consistent results since other scales may have different calibrations.

Manufacturers actually aim for the right mix of fat, sugar, and salt to produce what is called the **Bliss Point**. The point where these three elements meet, in perfect harmony, to provide the right amount of sweetness, saltiness, and fullness of overall taste.

**Body's Set Point:** Throughout a person's life, based on age and physical activity, a person's weight probably hovers around a number until a change in lifestyle, activity, or age, moves that set weight up or down.

**Calories:** This number represents the number of calories in 1 serving.

**Calorie Label:** The total calories, of all ingredients used in a recipe, divided by the number of portions, provides the calories for one serving.

**Daily Calorie Goal:** The total calories per day that will be eaten to maintain or reach a goal weight.

**Daily Quotient:** Daily Calories / Priorities = Balance

**Daily Eating Event:** This can be a specific food, number of alcoholic drinks, or a specific meal that will be the caloric priority for the day. This event allows for planning to stay within the daily calorie goal.

**Deadweight Calories:** These calories are neither needed or easily processed by the body, in a sedentary state, and can wreak havoc on the daily and weekly calorie goal.

**Empty Calories:** Calories that contain little or no nutritional value.

**EPOC** is the phenomenon known as **excess post** exercise **oxygen consumption**. The body will continue to burn calories at a higher metabolic rate for hours after an intense workout is finished.

**Excess of Quantity:** Consume more than is necessary, to enjoy the taste, and satisfy a craving or desire.

**High Calorie Obstacles:** Foods high in calories, fat, and carbohydrates, that can delay reaching a goal weight, or cause a backslide due to their universal appeal.

Two types of **Kryptonite:** What food or drink will absolutely cause a body to gain weight? What food or drink can a person not resist?

**Quality of Taste:** The enjoyment of the flavor and taste of food in a normal portion or small quantity.

**Serving Size:** A portion designated by the manufacturer. This may be the entire package or any of a number of units of measure, from grams, tablespoons, cups, pounds, ounces, or even a certain number of pieces.

**Servings Per Container:** This number designates how many servings in the specified serving size are in the entire package.

**Sweet Tooth:** A desire for confection after any meal.

**Yearly Cycle:** Every person that has struggled to maintain a goal weight has a yearly cycle. The cycle contains one or more periods where maintaining a goal weight is difficult or impossible.

**Zen:** The things that bring mind, body, and soul together as one.

# Website Reference Material

1. Mayo Clinic Staff. (2014,September 19). Metabolism and weight loss: How you burn calories. Retrieved from http://www.mayoclinic.org/healthy-lifestyle/weight-loss/in-depth/metabolism/art-20020046508

2. The best ways to boost your metabolism. Retrieved from http://www.health.com/health/gallery/0,,20306911,00.html

3. The Nutrition Source, What should I eat? Protein. Retrieved from https://www.hsph.harvard.edu/nutritionalsource/what-should-you-eat-/protein/

4. Jesse Szalay. (2015, August 25).What are carbohydrates? Retrieved from http://www.livescience.com/51976-carbohydrates.html

5. Types of Fats-Topic Overview. Retrieved from http://www.webmd.com/diet.guide/types-of-fats-topic-overview

6. Adda Bjarnadottir, MS. 11 Evidence-Based Health Benefits of Bananas. Retrieved from https://authoritynutrition.com/11-proven-benefits-of-bananas/

7. Bliss Point. Retrieved from https://en.m.wikipedia.org/wiki/Bliss_point_(food)

8. Honor Whiteman. (2015, October 28). Caffeine: How does it affect our health? Retrieved from http://www.medicalnewstoday.com/articles/271707.php

9. Elaine Magee, MPH, RD. The Best Bread: Tips for Buying Breads. Retrieved from http://www.webmd.com/food-recipes/features/the_best_ bread_tips_ for_ buying_ breads

10. 6 ways Cinnamon Can Aid Weight Loss. Retrieved from
http://idealbite.com/cinnamon-for-weight-loss/

11. How does the ocean affect climate? Retrieved from
http://oceanexplorer.noaa.gov/facts/climate.html

12. M. Gideon Hoyle. (2016, June 6). 3 Specific Uses of Enzymes in the
Human Body. Retrieved from
http://www.livestrong.com/article/508661-3-specific-uses-of-enzymes-
in-the-human-body/

13. Estimated Number of Animal and Plant Species on Earth. Retrieved
from http://www.factmonster.com/ipka/A0934288.html